CHRISTIAN HEALING

CHRISTIAN HEALING

Everyday Questions and Straightforward Answers

Mike Endicott

Terra Nova Publications

First published by Terra Nova Publications, 2004

*Published in Great Britain by
Terra Nova Publications
PO Box 2400, Bradford on Avon, Wiltshire BA15 2YN*

ISBN 1 90194 929 X

*Printed in Great Britain
by Bookmarque Ltd, Croydon*

Contents

PART THREE: QUESTIONS ON THE WAY

PART FOUR: MORE BIBLICAL ISSUES

PART FIVE: PASTORAL AND PRACTICAL

Introduction

1. What is Christian healing?

Christian healing is what happens when Christians minister in Jesus' name, enabling people to receive restoration to health of body or mind through God's great love and mercy. This restoration of health is part of what is meant by the 'abundant life', which Jesus promised.

Before the coming of Christ, the Jewish people already knew that God was a restorer, and that his will was to bring to fulfilment the work of restoration. The Hebrew prophets foretold the coming of the Messiah, and it was revealed that he would be one who heals:

> Surely he took up our infirmities
> and carried our sorrows,
> yet we considered him stricken by God,
> smitten by him, and afflicted.
> But he was pierced for our transgressions,
> he was crushed for our iniquities;
> the punishment that brought us
> peace was upon him,
> and by his wounds we are healed.
>
> *Isaiah 53:4–5*

For three years, the priests and religious leaders rejected Jesus. Many despised him, but others received him and became his disciples. Betrayed by one of his own disciples, denied by another, and abandoned by all, he died. Never has anyone else achieved so much nor been subjected to so much contempt. Jesus, the eternal Son of God, took upon himself on the cross all the evil that was due by justice to the entire human race—to Adam and all his descendants, including ourselves, so that anyone who believes in Jesus Christ and receives him as Saviour and Lord may receive all the blessings of God's kingdom, rather than eternal death. This is the 'great exchange'.

We may divide the great exchange of Calvary into five sub–sections, thus making it a little easier for us to grasp its amazing extent. Firstly, our punishment was exchanged for God's peace. As he died, Jesus bore the punishment that was due to us for our transgressions and all our iniquities, our acts of rebellion against God's laws. All the punishment for every sinful act committed by every member of the entire human race was brought onto Jesus. The blessing now available, the alternative to eternal punishment, is summed up in the word 'peace'. In place of punishment, there is peace for the believer. Secondly, our poverty has been exchanged for God's riches: that poverty with which we were cursed in our disobedience.

> Because you did not serve the LORD your God joyfully and gladly in the time of prosperity, therefore in hunger and thirst, in nakedness and dire poverty, you will serve the enemies the LORD sends against you. He will put an iron yoke on your neck until he has destroyed you.
>
> *Deuteronomy 28:47–48*

Jesus took our poverty onto the cross so that we might have his riches. He was hungry, not having eaten for almost twenty–four hours. He himself said, "I thirst." He was naked, for the soldiers had taken all his clothes for themselves, casting lots for his seamless robe. He was totally bereft of everything, a picture of total poverty, exhausting the curse. Jesus, who was rich with heaven's riches, became poor on the cross so that we might in turn share in his riches. Thirdly, Jesus has exchanged our mortality for a share in his immortality.

> But we see Jesus, who was made a little lower than the angels, now crowned with glory and honour because he suffered death, so that by the grace of God he might taste death for everyone.
>
> *Hebrews 2:9*

Fourthly, through Jesus we have been offered his righteousness instead of our own efforts to be holy.

> For we know that our old self was crucified with him so that the body of sin might be done away with, that we should no longer be slaves to sin....
>
> *Romans 6:6*

Fifthly, our sicknesses and pains have been taken on the cross so that we might receive healing through Jesus' wounds. He suffered terrible flogging and the imposition of the crown of thorns, and was crucified. As those terrible wounds were inflicted, so the covenant remedy for the pains and sicknesses of the whole human race was given. In accepting those things, he has made complete provision for our healing. On the cross was a bleeding, torn, wounded body, bereft of all things, who took upon himself the punishment due for all our sins, as well as our curses and our poverty —all this so that we might be forgiven and reconciled with the Father, as well as inheriting his peace, receiving healing, deliverance from evil, and abundant life. So Jesus said, "It is finished."

Salvation includes all of these five benefits obtained for the believer by Jesus Christ on the cross. We receive this salvation by the grace (free gift) of God, through faith in Jesus which we need to confess with our lips and believe in our hearts. He bore our griefs and carried our sorrows, and, as Isaiah prophesied, **by his wounds we are healed**—Jesus was physically wounded so that we might be healed. So the heavenly Father, our healer, sent his Son, Jesus, to earth, revealing his nature—and we saw the healing of the sick. Just as it is God's nature to love, so it is his nature to heal. He came as suffering servant and Saviour, yet everything was placed under his feet. Jesus will return and be seen by all as Lord of lords and King of kings. In the meantime, he has commissioned his people—the church, the company of believers—to preach the saving gospel and to heal the sick.

> Everything flows from how we learn the patience to stand under the Cross of Jesus, because when we are there we see what he sees, the infinite glory and love of the Father. That is where the healing fountains start.
>
> *Archbishop Rowan Williams*

We may wonder how Christian healing works. How can it be that God intervenes miraculously? Quite simply, though we do not understand *how* he does it, we know that our supernatural God is the Creator of the universe—from the largest galaxy to the most infinitesimal subatomic charge or particle. He brought into being and sustains in being all matter that exists; so nothing is impossible for him. Without him, nothing would exist at all: no universe; nothing! It is hardly surprising, then, that he who is Creator of all has the power to change things in this world that he created.

Part One

Why Sickness?

2. Am I sick for a reason?

On one level, of course, medical experts will sometimes be able to provide 'reasons' why an illness occurs: genetic or environmental factors may be involved; there may be a variety of physical causes at work in and upon a person. But people often ask this on a 'spiritual' level. They wonder whether, in some mysterious sense, there is a supernatural reason for their sickness. Sadly, many people have a sub-Christian notion of who God is and what his revealed will is, so in the course of this book we will be examining quite a few of the misunderstandings that arise. We will try to sort some of them out and begin to make sense of it all.

This question sometimes arises because of a widespread misunderstanding of the Book of Job. Some suggest that God made Job ill in order to bring him to his knees—in order that a fresh relationship between them could begin. On that view, God had a purpose in seeing Job become sick, and it would then follow that we, too, can believe that we are experiencing sickness sent by God for our own ultimate good. However this is a serious misapplication of the Job account. God has revealed his nature throughout both the Old and New

Testaments as the One who heals; his will is to heal. There are countless passages that bear this out.

Importantly, God did in fact heal Job—a point which seems to escape most people who know of his story. In the end, Job lived to be a hundred and forty years old and was greatly blessed by God after his time of sickness. He experienced a double restoration of all the things that he had temporarily lost at the hands of the devil. Satan robbed, killed, destroyed and afflicted, but God healed, delivered and restored. So even if we do (mistakenly) think that our own sickness is some sort of act of God (or approved by God), we should still expect that the final result will be healing and health rather than further sickness or death. When someone known to us falls ill and dies, it should be very clear to the rest of us that they had not been experiencing anything that we might loosely describe as a Job–like experience, otherwise they would have recovered! We can also reflect on the fact that Job was only ill for a small part of his life (widely agreed upon to be less than a year of it). Less than one percent of Job's life is described in detail in the Book of Job, so the wrong–headed idea that God wishes someone to be ill for long periods finds no support. We are not to suppose that God prolongs the sickness of the righteous for his own purposes. Above all, such a mistaken view of God, his will and the way he acts, conflicts with all that Jesus Christ revealed to us about God's heart for healing.

There are always reasons of various kinds why we fall ill, but the cause of your illness is never God.

3. Is illness some sort of punishment? Have I done something wrong? Do I deserve what is happening to me?

Even when there is true expectancy of healing (not just a belief that miracles do sometimes happen), it is sometimes the case that little or no improvement is visible after prayer. Then there may arise a tension in faith, which can go on to become a crisis of faith. Other issues may begin to come to the surface.

At that point it is sometimes said, "God is punishing me", or, "I deserve what I am getting", or, "Perhaps God won't heal me because I've been working too hard and not taking proper care of myself, smoking too much, eating either too much or all the wrong things." Or it may be that friends are trying to help by suggesting that some sin or some backsliding, or a period of irregular attendance at church, may be the problem.

In time the crisis passes. Sometimes a 'blockage' is revealed and dealt with. The supplicant finds, or has restored, a simple faith in Christ as healer. A properly equipped minister can often help the supplicant deal with the crises and blockages by explaining the nature of the Father, as revealed through Jesus in the Gospels. As the word of God is spoken and received, the supplicant begins to be able to receive healing much more easily.

We speak to the sick about the nature of Jesus. He shows us what the love, joy, peace, patience, kindness, goodness, faithfulness, gentleness and self-control of which we learn in Galatians chapter five really look like. The love of Jesus; the compassion of Jesus; the mercy of Jesus —all reveal to us the heart of the Father towards us. Those whom Jesus healed in his earthly ministry were not perfect by any means. They simply had faith, or others had faith, for their healing. The supplicant may need to be reminded that '...he should ask

God, who gives generously to all without finding fault....' (See James 1:5.) Isaiah described in advance what was going to happen to Jesus. (See Isaiah 53:1–6). Clearly, any punishment that is due to us has already been dealt with by God: his wrath against us has been exhausted on the cross.

The idea that God wants to strike people with sickness in order to punish them is foreign to the New Testament. Of course, we sometimes become aware that an illness we contract has been due wholly or partly to some sin or foolishness for which we bear some responsibility. If that is revealed to us, then we do need to repent, and God will forgive us. But 'sin hunting' and 'working down checklists' is not how the healing ministry should be conducted. The Holy Spirit will do any convicting that is necessary. In the end, nothing can separate us from the love of God in Christ Jesus.

A common mistake is to think that God may be using or prolonging sickness as a mysterious form of discipline. After all, we reason, Scripture does teach that God disciplines his children. A more careful reading of Hebrews 12:7, though, reveals that it is hardship, not illness, that may be used by God to discipline us, and this would be done in the same way that a good earthly father might discipline us, and for the same good, loving motive. Jesus explained that not even a human father would give his son a snake instead of a fish, nor a scorpion instead of an egg. (See Luke 11:11–12). God really does love us as his children. He does not make you ill!

To summarise: firstly, it is extremely unlikely that your illness is a punishment. When you received Jesus, his work on the cross included taking the punishment for your sin; secondly, if you contributed to your sickness by your own wrong actions, you can repent and be forgiven and restored; thirdly, it makes little sense in the healing ministry to talk of what we *deserve,* for all good things are in any case the free gifts of our Creator and Redeemer; the bad things that affect us result from the disorder that flows from Adam's first disobedience, and from Satan's malign influence.

4. Why did God allow me or a member of my family to get ill?

We can see in the answer to question 3 that this is not an issue of punishment. God's will for his people is that they should have abundant life, not condemnation.

> For God so loved the world that he gave his one and only Son, that whoever believes in him shall not perish but have eternal life. For God did not send his Son into the world to condemn the world, but to save the world through him. Whoever believes in him is not condemned...
>
> *John 3:16–18a*

Behind the question is, often, a sense of unfairness. Sickness sometimes seems to us to be so random. So the age–old question haunts many who suffer: "Why me?" Add the statement, "It's all so unfair" and we touch something of the rawness of life. But please remember this: God is not the author of sickness; he did not place sickness on you or your loved ones. Sickness itself is the outworking of a kind of enemy activity which is one of the many consequences of the Fall. Do not blame God for what the devil has brought about, nor for the harm mankind has done to itself. God is not the cause of any ill–health or injury; he is the one who rescues us from sickness—who heals our diseases.

It is somewhat misleading to reduce this issue to 'God's permissive will' because sickness is not what God wills at all. His revealed will is both to heal us and to draw us to himself and to bring us into his kingdom of love. Had he made mankind to be merely automatons, pre–programmed never to make the wrong choice to sin, never to have the choice of disobeying or obeying, there would have been no Fall and no sickness either—but nor would there have been any possibility of a response of love for God. If God were to make man in his own image and to be capable of a love response to the Creator, then man had to be endowed with kinds of freedom that could be open to misuse.

So it is most helpful to see an individual's sickness not as imposed by God, but rather as an outworking of living in a fallen world, in which mankind's own disobedience has all sorts of negative consequences. We are affected not only by our own sins, but by the sinful acts of others, the general sinfulness of mankind and the demonic activity to which man's disobedience has opened so many doors.

God's answer to this mess which we and the rest of the human race have made was to reveal his nature as the healer, deliverer and Redeemer of all who turn to him. With God, fresh starts are available. Jesus came to destroy the works of the devil (including all forms of ill–health), to bind up the broken–hearted and to set captives free. We enter into all this, which Jesus won for us by grace, through faith in him, believing in our hearts and confessing with our lips.

5. But what about life–threatening diseases?

This is a question which deeply affects our expectancy of God—that expectancy which acts as a 'lightning rod' in the heavenly places. This 'lightning rod' has to poke up just a little above the roof top, and fears that illnesses are life–threatening may detract from an undoubting trust in Jesus to solve the problem. When people hear the medical diagnosis that a disease is incurable or life–threatening, terror and sadness may come in and become a weighty burden. Then it is vital to cling to God's promises—if only as a man clings to a tuft of grass on the cliff edge over which he has just fallen. Our hope may become thinner as time wears on, and our child–like expectancy that God is going to heal us smaller than a mustard seed. Our natural reaction to the threat of a dreadful disability is to lower our lightning rods of faith expectancy.

From the point of view of the minister, the more threatening the illness, the harder we tend to feel we will have to work in prayer, fasting and in ministry. As many die, despite all our efforts, we become confirmed in our view that some things are going to be harder work for God than others. Cancer is a much bigger nut to crack than a passing headache, we suppose. Here we can see yet more forces at work that would lower our expectancy. The more the minister worries about his own role in the healing, the more he wrongly supposes that he or she carries responsibility for the process. The greater this assumption, the less reliance is placed on God—and the mustard seed may become smaller still.

However, this measuring of the severity of an illness flows from our own experience and ideas, rather than the truth about what God can do. The medical profession might, on the evidence of their research, classify some diseases as incurable, but in the kingdom of God no disease presents the Lord with greater difficulty than another. We tend to think about our past experience of prayer, and the levels of apparent success and failure we have seen, as the measure of God's power and willingness to see healing done. But the revelation of God the Father comes only through Jesus, so to really know God's will and power we must watch the ministry of Jesus in the Gospels—and we see there that he never failed to heal anyone on the grounds that the problem was too hard for him. People's unbelief could be a hindrance, but Jesus never let anyone down who came to him for healing on the grounds that their problems were too huge, or that God wanted them to suffer or to die before their time. Power was coming out of Jesus and healing all who came to him. The same is true today. Jesus was raised from the dead; he is alive and he is the same tomorrow and today as he was then, in the Gospel accounts of healing. Power is still flowing from him for all of us. Moreover, he has given power, authority and a command to his disciples to heal the sick, with the promise that they will do even greater things.

> He went down with them and stood on a level place. A large crowd of his disciples was there and a great number of people from all over Judea, from Jerusalem, and from the coast of Tyre and Sidon, who had come to hear him and to be healed of their diseases. Those troubled by evil spirits were cured, and the people all tried to touch him, because power was coming from him and healing them all.
>
> *Luke 6:17–19*

Part Two

Faith in God

6. How should I approach God for my own healing?

To seek our own healing from God, first and foremost we need to believe that it is his will to see *everyone* receive healing who comes to him. We must expect it to happen. The sum 'our faith minus our doubts' has to leave us with a 'mustard seed' of faith that healing is for us before we are in a place to begin to receive. Then we need the persistence and the humility to reach out for him, and to keep reaching out, until we receive what he has for us. We need to walk humbly with him, putting aside our questions, our doubts about God's power and love, and our criticisms of any abuses we may have seen, and fall on our faces before the Lord.

Secondly, we need to know and believe ourselves to be in the presence of God, not merely as one might entertain or give credence to a theological concept, but because we are aware of the awesome and almost tangible nature of his presence with us. This supernatural reality is expressed powerfully in this passage, providing us with a clear 'window':

> After this I looked and there before me was a great multitude that no one could count, from every nation,

tribe, people and language, standing before the throne and in front of the Lamb. They were wearing white robes and were holding palm branches in their hands. And they cried out in a loud voice: "Salvation belongs to our God, who sits on the throne, and to the Lamb."

All the angels were standing around the throne and around the elders and the four living creatures. They fell down on their faces before the throne and worshipped God, saying:

"Amen! Praise and glory and wisdom and thanks and honour and power and strength be to our God for ever and ever. Amen!"

Revelation 7:9–12

In the presence of God, how does one pray? How does one express needs to the Lamb on the throne? Amongst the holy throng how do we even open our mouths? The awesome presence of God is such that we can do nothing but worship him.

So do not worry, saying, 'What shall we eat?' or 'What shall we drink?' or 'What shall we wear?' For the pagans run after all these things, and your heavenly Father knows that you need them. But seek first his kingdom and his righteousness, and all these things will be given to you as well.

Matthew 6:31–33

How should we approach God for our own healing? With expectant and child–like hearts, as out of our mouths comes worship, thanksgiving and praise.

7. Do I have enough faith to be healed?

Most likely, yes. Many Christians who have not yet received the promised healing feel rejected by God, even let down by him in their hour of need. This idea that there has been a 'failure' to meet their need may then turn into self–blame. The self–accusation emerges from the feeling that one does not have enough faith. Sufferers sometimes say that they will not attend healing services because they do not have the faith for that sort of thing.

In the context of Christian healing it is not right to think of our lack of faith, as we understand the meaning of that word today, as being a faulty belief system which will turn God away in judgement, withdrawing his healing hand. Faith, when simply described as the supplicant's belief in Jesus as Son of God, and belief in his virgin birth, his death and resurrection, is not in question here. It is not lack of such credal faith that limits our ability to receive healing, but rather our lack of simple and child–like expectancy that he will do it.

All the philosophical, cynical, sceptical and scientific reasoning that we use to avoid or bend the simple truth about God's healing heart makes many of us, to use the biblical term, 'double–minded' about such things. On the one hand, we believe in Jesus as Saviour and accept that he is quite capable of doing healing miracles, but on the other hand we have grave doubts about his readiness to do it to us, now, and we feel that there are so many unanswered questions. This puts us in two minds. We have sufficient faith and yet we also have doubts—the word 'doubt' being translated from a Greek word meaning 'alternative viewpoint'. In this doubting frame of mind we appear like a man trying to row a boat along a waterway with an oar (his faith) in one hand and a canoe paddle (alternative views) clasped firmly in the other. He is actually going around in circles, not because of any weakness in the oar but because of the use of a paddle in the other hand. His rowing is distinctly 'double–minded'! He has one mindset that tells him that Jesus healed everyone who came to him and is the same good God today as he was yesterday; but in another, concurrent, mindset he has his 'Ah, but...'s. Unless he stops being double–minded, he cannot really expect to get anywhere fast!

> Jesus replied, "I tell you the truth, if you have faith and do not doubt, not only can you do what was done to the fig tree, but also you can say to this mountain, 'Go, throw yourself into the sea,' and it will be done. If you believe, you will receive whatever you ask for in prayer."
>
> *Matthew 21:21–22*

See also No. 24 *Could God be delaying his healing?*

8. Where do I get the faith to see healing?

Whatever we say about faith being important for seeing healing miracles happen (as taught by Jesus), we should always remember he also revealed that we need only to have a 'mustard seed' amount of it. Such is the grace of God that this really is sufficient. Faith like this is a deep, uncluttered and child–like personal trust in the total reliability of Jesus—the same miracle–working Jesus whom we see in the Gospels. The New Testament lists faith among the nine gifts of the Spirit; and tells us all that we have been given a measure of faith, and that faith is a fruit of the Holy Spirit. In a special way, the Holy Spirit grows faith, as fruit, in the lives of very human believers. The Bible also makes it clear that it is something we have to exercise, because Jesus tells us to 'have faith'; not to doubt but to believe.

The growth of the fruit of faith, as with all the fruit of the Holy Spirit, makes Christian believers become more as God intended; more like Christ. The Christian life is marked by that ongoing process. This is faith in action:

> Is any one of you sick? He should call the elders of the church to pray over him and anoint him with oil in the name of the Lord. And the prayer offered in faith will make the sick person well; the Lord will raise him up. If he has sinned, he will be forgiven.
>
> *James 5:14–15*

So how do we obtain enough faith to see people healed? The first step is to begin to hear the word of God, for faith comes by hearing that word.

> Consequently, faith comes from hearing the message, and the message is heard through the word of Christ.
>
> *Romans 10:17*

So the way to perform healing and miracles, as the apostles did, is to see Jesus in the Gospels as the perfect revelation of the Father's will to heal, watch him working through the hands of others in the church, and operating in the faith that comes from hearing, believing and applying the anointed word of God. When the disciples asked Jesus how they might perform miracles, his answer was to focus their beliefs.

> Then they asked him, "What must we do to do the works God requires?"
>
> Jesus answered, "The work of God is this: to believe in the one he has sent."
>
> *John 6:28*

9. What is the 'prayer offered in faith'?

> And the prayer offered in faith will make the sick person well; the Lord will raise him up. If he has sinned, he will be forgiven.
>
> *James 5:15*

Does this phrase 'prayer offered in faith' mean that we should wait until we have some sudden or great influx of faith that assures us so mightily of an imminent healing that we have almost to do nothing but stand and wait for it? Or, on the other hand, do we speak out the prayer of faith when we have understood in our minds that Jesus heals and that we have authority over sickness and disease? If we then speak the words 'Be healed!', will it happen for us? We may look very foolish if it does not! How do we pray an effective prayer of faith? How do we do the works that God intends us to do? We should forget what is in our minds and consider what is in our hearts. In John's Gospel we find the followers of Jesus facing the same misunderstandings. Jesus told his disciples that the work of God is to believe in the one he has sent (see John 6:28–29). In other words, we can be used by God, through the power of the Holy Spirit, to heal the sick if we simply believe that Jesus did do it, that he can do it and that he will do it. If we trust enough to rely totally on him then we begin to pray in faith, whatever the form of prayer we use. But how to deepen our trust? One most important way is to move more deeply into the heart knowledge that Father God wills healing for everyone.

> Jesus answered, "I am the way and the truth and the life. No one comes to the Father except through me. If you really knew me, you would know my Father as well. From now on, you do know him and have seen him."
>
> *John 14:6–7*

Here Jesus is impressing on Philip that we can see the Father heart of God if we watch his words and works. In verse eight Philip says, "Lord, show us the Father and that will be enough for us." Philip is struggling to understand.

Then Jesus answers:

> "Don't you know me, Philip, even after I have been among you such a long time? Anyone who has seen me has seen the Father. How can you say, 'Show us the Father'? Don't you believe that I am in the Father, and that the Father is in me? The words I say to you are not just my own. Rather, it is the Father, living in me, who is doing his work...."

Jesus points out that it is the Father, living in him, who is doing his work; nowadays it is Jesus living within *us* who is doing the work. So what exactly do we have to believe if we want to pray the prayer of faith and heal the sick as did Jesus and the apostles? In verse eleven, Jesus continues, "Believe me when I say that I am in the Father and the Father is in me; or at least believe on the evidence of the miracles themselves." So the fuel for the prayer of faith is our believing that Jesus, by doing miracles of healing, is showing us the 'heartbeat' of God.

Amazing things will start to happen if we really get this under our belt: that the heart of God is to see *everyone* who comes to him healed. In vv. 12–14, Jesus assures us:

> "I tell you the truth, anyone who has faith in me will do what I have been doing. He will do even greater things than these, because I am going to the Father. And I will do whatever you ask in my name, so that the Son may bring glory to the Father. You may ask me for anything in my name, and I will do it."

So there is no method of praying—no prescriptive answer—only a compassionate ache for those who suffer, and a concrete trust in the will of God to heal. There are often times when we cannot pray in words at all, nor even feel that we can pray in any way as we ought to. However, our inarticulate longings for a more abundant life for the supplicant in front of us are the Spirit's intercessions on our behalf. These silent yearnings are audible to God who searches all our hearts, and are both intelligible and acceptable to him because they are the voice of his Spirit. It is, after all, in accordance with his will that the Spirit should intercede for us.

Jesus himself never *prayed for* the sick; he simply gave healing to them. He lived his life in complete dependence upon the Father, as we all ought to do. To appear before him, to stand in the kingdom in his healing presence, may often limit the minister entirely to worship. This can be what happens as the 'prayer of faith' takes place. It is then that the person ministering knows exactly where they are and what is around them, and is reacting in the only way that they can to the presence of God.

For further reading on this matter see No. 7 *Do I have enough faith to be healed?*

10. What is the power?

The power to heal is not a thing but a person. The apostles, and the early church disciples, did not believe that the risen, glorified Jesus was passive or inactive; on the contrary, they knew that he was at work in his body, the church. In their experience he was powerfully changing lives. Signs and wonders were following the preaching of the good news. In the beginning, John the Baptist had been teaching his disciples to expect from Jesus the baptism of the Spirit—not of water only, as in his own baptismal rite. Before his death on the cross, Jesus continued to fill his disciples' minds with the expectation of this gift of the Spirit; and, some ten days after Jesus disappeared from their sight, that Spirit had come in power upon them. This same Holy Spirit was the Spirit of God, and also, and therefore, the Spirit of Jesus. Jesus could not be thought of merely as a perfect past example, or a remote Lord, but an inward presence and power. World history shows us that the impact of mere examples, whether they be people or an experience of some massive event, becomes more and more feeble as time progresses. The example of Jesus, however, had become something much more than a memory. He who had, in the past, taught them how to live in the kingdom, was alive in the heavenly places and was working within them by his Spirit, to extend that very same kingdom. And the result? There is now great power for those of us who believe.

> I keep asking that the God of our Lord Jesus Christ, the glorious Father, may give you the Spirit of wisdom and revelation, so that you may know him better. I pray also that the eyes of your heart may be enlightened in order that you may know the hope to which he has called you, the riches of his glorious inheritance in the saints, and his incomparably great power for us who believe. That power is like the working of his mighty strength, which he exerted in Christ when he raised him from the dead and seated him at his right hand in the heavenly realms, far above all rule and authority, power and dominion, and every title that can be given, not only in the present age but also in the one to come. And God placed all things under his feet and appointed him to be head over everything for the church, which is his body, the fullness of him who fills everything in every way.
>
> *Ephesians 1:17–19*

And how should we think of Jesus within? He is the Son of God, the Creator of the universe who makes all things new; the one who healed everyone who asked him, because he knew that it is the will of the Father that all who respond to this Jesus should have salvation. And this salvation includes physical and emotional healing for all who respond like little children to the Good News.

11. How much can we rely on God to do it?

The miracles of Jesus and the benefits of his death on the cross are a focused reflection of God's heart for his hurting children. We are totally dependent on him for the power to heal, but God has decided already what his will is on the matter; and that will is clearly revealed in the character and ministry of his Son, Jesus. He was always willing to heal all, and this consistent disposition is a reflection of the Father's heart towards all of us.

> While Jesus was in one of the towns, a man came along who was covered with leprosy. When he saw Jesus, he fell with his face to the ground and begged him, "Lord, if you are willing, you can make me clean."
>
> Jesus reached out his hand and touched the man. "I am willing," he said. "Be clean!" And immediately the leprosy left him.
>
> *Luke 5:12 –15*

It was always so. Even before New Testament times, before God was fully revealed to us in Jesus, the people of God always knew that he was an unlimited healer:

Praise the LORD, O my soul;
all my inmost being, praise his holy name.
Praise the LORD, O my soul,
and forget not all his benefits—
who forgives all your sins
and heals all your diseases,
who redeems your life from the pit
and crowns you with love and compassion,
who satisfies your desires with good things
so that your youth is renewed like the eagle's.
The LORD works righteousness
and justice for all the oppressed.

Psalm 103:1–6

If we believe that we must prayerfully find out about God's will from healing situation to healing situation, then we have not seen clearly enough that God has already revealed his will in his Son. Anyone thinking that they must determine the will of God afresh as to whether he will or not heal the supplicant will have problems maintaining any sort of consistent ministry of healing the sick and injured. The implicit belief that God's will might change, depending on the individual case, only serves to produce doubt in the hearts of both the minister and the supplicant, interfering with the consistent flow of good results.

We need to cultivate a much more Christ–centred view of healing. We can be assured that all who came to Jesus received from him, and we must be alive to the fact that God's will on the matter has been settled in heaven and revealed in his word.

12. Does God need a faith environment into which he can heal?

For the purposes of healing the sick and injured we may define a 'faith environment' as being a meeting together of hearts who trust in Jesus as Lord, Saviour and healer. Jesus is the perfecter of our faith and the perfect revelation of the Father. If we ask 'Does God...?' we can always ask 'Did Jesus...?' —and arrive at an accurate answer. This may, at first glance, lead to the most child–like theology, but this is infinitely preferable for those who seek to heal and be healed. Much complex theology sows doubt.

There are certainly specific occasions in the Gospel accounts of Jesus healing the sick and injured where Jesus points out to the healed supplicant that it is their faith that has made them well again. There are also a number of occasions when Jesus checks in advance to make sure sufficient faith (a mustard seed) is present. An example of this approach can be found in Matthew 9:28.

> When he had gone indoors, the blind men came to him, and he asked them, "Do you believe that I am able to do this?"
>
> "Yes, Lord," they replied.

There are both general and specific miracle workings recorded in Jesus' ministry where the seed of faith already existed and may well have been the factor that drew the supplicant to Jesus for healing in the first place.

> Then they came to Jericho. As Jesus and his disciples, together with a large crowd, were leaving the city, a blind man, Bartimaeus (that is, the Son of Timaeus), was sitting by the roadside begging. When he heard that it

> was Jesus of Nazareth, he began to shout, "Jesus, Son of David, have mercy on me!"
>
> *Mark 10:46–47*

There are also occasions when miracles were worked where there is no specific evidence that any faith existed at all. There are a number of instances where the faith of family and friends was present, but others where as far as we know it was completely absent, such as the healing of the man who had been born blind. (See John 9:1–7). There we have some interesting discussion on the subject of sin (Jesus made it clear that the blindness was not caused by sin in the man or his parents), but there is no hint that the blind man came into the situation with any faith, nor that any was raised up in him by listening to the conversation going on around him.

However, the most quoted passage on the subject of the need for the presence of faith is to be found in Matthew 13:54a, 57 and 58.

> Coming to his hometown, he began teaching the people in their synagogue, and they were amazed.... And they took offence at him.
>
> But Jesus said to them, "Only in his hometown and in his own house is a prophet without honour."
>
> And he did not do many miracles there because of their lack of faith.

Jesus is not always depicted as having to create a faith environment in the supplicants: sometimes the people brought one with them. Accounts of healing where there is little or no evidence of any faith environment at all are comparatively rare. We might be well advised to consider in this context the nature of the culture in which we are attempting to minister. Some churches would need no faith building, whilst some may need extensive teaching on the kingdom of God to have their expectancy sufficiently raised. Even within the congregation of expectant churches there will be those who would love to be healed but whose doubts will limit their own openness to receive.

On a much larger scale, the level of the general 'water table of expectancy' among Christians can vary considerably between nations—levels of basic scepticism being higher or lower among different national cultures. Taking all this into consideration, it may always be wise to spend some time in lifting the expectancy of those who would come to Jesus. In view of the growth of complex healing theology over the centuries, and the church's reliance on its own experience to prove the will of God, simple and Christ–centred faith building is always a good thing to do. The gift of faith then flows into the people through that teaching, and their faith expectancy enables them to receive healing.

13. What must I believe in to see healing?

First of all we should define what is meant here by a miracle. We might say that God has always been turning water into wine. He created vines and the soil in which they grow. He has organised our climate so that rain falls on the vine, is sucked up into the plant and fills the budding grapes. Collected by men and fermented by God–created processes, wine emerges, to the enjoyment of man and the glory of God. A miracle is seen to have been done when God supernaturally speeds up the process, as Jesus did at the wedding at Cana. Within our bodies we have a number of systems ready–built to provide healing forces within us. Where these are damaged or prove inadequate, and God is involved through prayer, such systems are supernaturally speeded up, to give us a healing miracle. Jesus consistently refers to such miracles as 'works', the inference being that his healing miracles were the work of God, the sort of thing that happens regularly and fruitfully in the kingdom of God. There were many in Jesus' time, as there are today, who sought to work miracles.

> Then they asked him, "What must we do to do the works God requires?"
>
> Jesus answered, "The work of God is this: to believe in the one he has sent."
>
> *John 6:28–29*

What does it really mean —to 'believe in...'? If it means merely that we must have head knowledge that Jesus is the Christ, a person of the Holy Trinity, subject of the virgin birth, resurrection and ascension, and that he once had the power to heal (and still does) then the entire Christian church would find healing the sick an easy thing to do. Many do believe those things. What really matters is our relationship of trust with him. Justification by grace through faith (or coming into a right relationship with God) is not something that happens by virtue of our believing in the *doctrine* of justification by faith; but, rather, because we have come to the cross and received Jesus as Saviour and Lord, and been born again by the Spirit of God. So we begin to love the Lord our God with all our heart and mind and strength. Similarly, we are not healed simply because we believe Jesus was a healer and is still alive today. We come in love and simple, child–like trust to our Father in heaven who loves us and whom we love. Expectancy in our hearts that Jesus can be trusted to let mercy flow every time—without exception—into all who ask, is a working belief in the healing context. The understanding that God does not make individual decisions about healing which may vary from one person to another has to sink very deep into the hearts of all involved. We have to believe in the Jesus of the Gospels, the totally reliable one, and not some other concept of Jesus who has to be somehow persuaded by clever, well thought out prayers, sent up to heaven by 'experts'. We have to believe that God's will is for the healing of all who ask us to minister it in the name of his Son.

These concepts are not necessarily easy to grasp or apply, and the disciples found the task daunting. We can read about Philip's struggle to understand in John 14:6ff.

See No. 9 *What is the prayer offered in faith?*

14. Why is our faith, our believing trust, so precious to God?

Why does God require expectancy and trust (faith) from us when his power is present to heal? Why does he need this mustard seed? Can't he do it anyway?

Underlying this sort of query there is another question widely and silently held in the hearts of many Christians: If God is really good, and all love, then why does he not simply act sovereignly and remove all suffering from the planet? Why does he demand faith first?

> Then Jesus told him [Thomas], "Because you have seen me, you have believed; blessed are those who have not seen and yet have believed."
>
> *John 20:29*

But why are they blessed any more than anyone else? Because faith expectancy pleases him. Why did Jesus constantly major on faith having such an important role in our receiving healing? Because looking for him in our troubles is our reaction to his love for us. Love demands a response. Any one of us who comes to the resurrected Lord to receive healing must somehow demonstrate to him that we completely believe he exists and rewards those of us who seriously seek him out in our weakness. If we press up into him then he presses down into us. This is the dynamic by which actual, holy power comes across the veil between heaven and earth.

> Now faith is being sure of what we hope for and certain of what we do not see. This is what the ancients were commended for.
>
> By faith we understand that the universe was formed at God's command, so that what is seen was not made out of what was visible.
>
> By faith Abel offered God a better sacrifice than Cain did. By faith he was commended as a righteous man, when God spoke well of his offerings. And by faith he still speaks, even though he is dead.
>
> By faith Enoch was taken from this life, so that he did not experience death; he could not be found, because God had taken him away. For before he was taken, he was commended as one who pleased God. And without faith it is impossible to please God, because anyone who comes to him must believe that he exists and that he rewards those who earnestly seek him.
>
> *Hebrews 11:1–6*

We can let our faith in Jesus Christ take hold of us but we cannot take hold of him. We may love to go so far as to sit on his knee but, when we do so, we will not be able to keep our feet off the ground for long, because the strains and stresses of the world bring restricting feelings, like a sort of cramp on our faith. All we can do is hold out a lame faith to Jesus like a beggar holding out a stump instead of a whole arm and cry, "Lord Jesus, work a miracle!"

15. Which of us has to have the faith to see healing: the minister, the supplicant or both?

The first thing to emphasise here is that by 'faith' we must mean 'expectancy'. We need to believe that it is God's will that everyone who comes to him for healing can be able to receive it. This is not quite the same as having faith that the healing will be received; but, rather, that the gift has already been provided for, as is shown both through the ministry of Jesus that revealed to us the Father's will and through his sacrifice for us on Calvary.

It is easy to misinterpret the word 'faith' in the context of Christian healing. In this situation there should be no question of examining the supplicant's own depth of faith relationship with God. How deeply the supplicant believes in Jesus as the Son of God, or how much they love him and rely on their having a relationship with him, is not the point for the person ministering and will not affect the supplicant's ability to receive healing. Nor is their understanding of doctrine of great importance here. Whilst Jesus did commend the faith of those sufferers who came to him believing, there were also occasions when others believed for the sick person. Healing could be ministered without preconditions! Does the teaching that healing depends on expectancy condemn those who are struggling with sickness? Absolutely not! All of us can obtain expectancy for healing or benefit from the faith expectancy of others. No-one need be left out.

If we wish to imitate our Lord's ministry of working miracles we must first teach the kingdom as he did. Many of the accounts of his miracles incorporate Jesus's teaching about how faith operates in the kingdom. Unhappily, some have been taught that expectancy is a static and a uniform thing, which we either 'have' or do not 'have'. However, the nature of true expectancy is that it constantly changes. It can grow, or decrease in strength, from day to day. Its level might be affected by our understanding of the Father's will for his sick children and by the clarity of our apprehension of the revelation of the love of God. It can be affected by our own state of mental and physical health and by the pressures of our personal situations. It can be affected by our theology and altered by our doubts. Our expectancy can be lifted through prayer and assiduous Bible study —as long as we are prepared to allow the Holy Spirit to adjust our thinking through such means. It is often found that sufficient expectancy for healing (a mustard seed) comes after hearing a confident proclamation of Jesus Christ as healer. In other words, it can be released. It might be that one day a minister or supplicant may have been weak in their expectancy, and the next day new levels of expectancy can be released from hearing some miraculous news about a relative or friend, or lifted by a presentation of the good news of the kingdom of God. A struggle today, issuing in the overthrowing of a theological doubt or a blocking mind–set, could release a new experience of healing tomorrow.

In other words, intellectual belief that Jesus did heal, and could heal today, does not affect the supplicant's ability to receive healing, however solid that belief may be. It is, rather, our simple, child–like expectancy of God that acts as a lightning conductor, helping us to see miraculous blessings. This expectancy comes from three sources, one or all of which may play a part during the ministry time. Firstly, it may be that the *supplicant* has all the expectancy needed to see themselves receive healing. Consider the case of a woman who had been subject to bleeding for twelve years:

> When she heard about Jesus, she came up behind him in the crowd and touched his cloak, because she thought, "If I just touch his clothes, I will be healed."
>
> Immediately her bleeding stopped and she felt in her body that she was freed from her suffering.
>
> *Mark 5:27–29*

Jesus, pointing, as he so often did, toward faith (which we are to understand as expectancy) as a determinate part of the healing process, said to her, "Daughter, your faith has healed you." We can conclude from Jesus' looking around to find out who had touched him that he did not know in advance that this would happen. The supplicant had all the expectancy —and enough to see healing flow. Secondly, it may be that the *minister* works a miracle, with no evident expectancy on the part of anyone else. A number of occasions recorded in the New Testament, especially those times when Jesus raised the dead, illustrate this possibility. It must be admitted that we do not often see healing miracles today when only the minister has faith expectancy for healing, but it can happen. Thirdly, there is corporate faith, the general level of expectancy in the room at the time, or in the *church*, as a ministry session begins. Of course God sees us all as individuals, with individual needs, but he also works through the gathered congregation, where two or three, or more, come together as part of his Son's Body in action.

> "Again, I tell you that if two of you on earth agree about anything you ask for, it will be done for you by my Father in heaven.
>
> For where two or three come together in my name, there am I with them."
>
> *Matthew 18:19–20*

God delights to work corporately through the church:

> His intent was that now, through the church, the manifold wisdom of God should be made known to the rulers and authorities in the heavenly realms, according to his eternal purpose which he accomplished in Christ Jesus our Lord.
>
> *Ephesians 3:10*

We should, then, expect to have expectancy but we should not expect to have to have all the expectancy! The ministry of healing is at its most effective when the minister, the supplicant and the gathered body are expectant and we are all in it together.

16. Should we really expect it to happen?

The problem with ministering healing is that, too often, we want to make it so much more complicated than it needs to be.

A lifetime's experience of unanswered prayer can so often be the thing that has led us away from *ministering* God's goodness into the 'easier' way of *interceding for it in the presence of the supplicant*, and that can be counter–productive because it raises doubt. This is not to criticise intercession as such; it is to say that it has largely become easier and safer, in front of the supplicant, to ask God for healing than it is to simply invite that person to step into the kingdom and receive what has already been given. Prayers of request in the presence of the supplicant may tend to give the impression that we presuppose God might not decide to heal on this occasion.

We develop all sorts of spurious reasons as to why God (sometimes) might not heal us; we play the 'blame game' of laying fault at God's door, or at the feet of the supplicant. All this so–called 'deeper understanding' of spiritual things (which is anything but), only leads to scepticism and doubt. Unbelief has all too often made the healing ministry of the Christian church into a hit–and–miss, 'religious' affair —trying it now and again, to see if God will 'do the business'.

But the fact is that wherever we see God at work in miraculous power we also see a childlike, simple, trusting expectancy into which the river of grace can flow.

> Jesus said, "Let the little children come to me, and do not hinder them, for the kingdom of heaven belongs to such as these."
>
> *Matthew 19:14*

When a meeting can take place between our simple, child–like expectancy and divine grace, it is as though heaven 'explodes'. We begin to see sick people healed in New Testament proportions.

This is not to think in a mechanistic way about divine, supernatural power. We are considering here the flow of mercy. Our intercessory requests may sometimes be hopeful, but are much less often marked by real, confident, trusting expectancy. There is incomparably great power available to us who believe, who are God's 'new creation'. We Christians have all been given the awesome and exciting responsibility of carrying the revealed word of God, together with the signs and wonders accompanying that word, to the world.

Every church, of course, in various ways, prays for those who are sick, but perhaps more out of Christian hope, love and duty than the real expectation that God will act, according to his promises. But add the particular ingredient of expectancy, along with persistence and humility, and those around the church begin to be healed of their sicknesses in numbers only dreamed of before.

But there is a supplementary question. Sometimes a person who really does have great expectancy that God heals, and wants to heal them, but who has not yet received healing, will ask: "How often should I ask for prayer?" The supplicant may (mistakenly) think that to repeat requests for healing for oneself is to display a lack of faith. The conviction may take root that God has heard our prayers, and is in the process of meshing our requests in with his great plans for the world, but that other things may have to drop into place first before the desired healing will come. To go on asking, they think, is to presume that God may not have heard, or at least not begun to do something about it. This logic is rarely applied to praying for others; in those cases, persistent and faithful praying is readily approved as being right. Consider again the teaching and example of Jesus. He consistently taught the need for continuous and persistent prayer until our object is achieved. Most healing is missed for want of such persistence. One of the major reasons for ineffective ministry is that we do not, or will not, press on into what has already been prepared for us. It is in persistence that we truly demonstrate our expectancy, the largest ingredient in our faith that opens us up to receiving healing. Nowadays, we expect instant solutions, and, as these rarely happen where expectancy is in short supply, we turn away with wistful thoughts of, 'Maybe one day....'

Having begun to sow seeds of doubt in our own minds, we become even less persistent and less expectant. The downward cycle of doubt into despair (or, worse, to the dismissal of the healing power of Jesus) begins. To counteract such negativity, if this is your problem, I suggest reading or re–reading the biblical account of Elisha's dealing with the Shunammite woman, recorded in 2 Kings 4. That incident, and the healing of Naaman in chapter five, provide powerful encouragement to us, demonstrating that God has always looked with favour on persistent faith and faithful action.

For further reading on this subject see No. 23 *Why is so much prayer apparently not answered?* and No. 41 *Does God raise the dead?* See also my book entitled *Heaven's Dynamite.*

Part Three

Questions on the Way

17. Why should we rely on God?

Our own experience of praying for those we care for is often erratic, and prayer sometimes seems to many to be a very unreliable form of treatment for sickness and injury, though they might not dare to admit that this is what they really think. So the mistake which is often made is subconsciously to assume that God himself is erratic and unreliable in fulfilling his promises. This only serves to breed more doubt, which in turn results in even less success at prayer.

It is not surprising that, today, even many of those who *theoretically* believe in healing have difficulty receiving. If only God's will to heal were taught amongst us with the same assurance as the truth that he is ready to forgive those who come to Jesus, then those hearing would receive healing much more easily.

The first principle to grasp is that the giving of healing by God and the receiving of it by human beings are two separate and distinct things. It is not the giving but the receiving which is problematical. We need to dwell deeply on the truth about the One who gives all good things. It was revealed in the Old Testament, long before God became man, that the Messiah would be a reliable healer.

Praise the LORD, O my soul;
and forget not all his benefits—
who forgives all your sins
and heals all your diseases....

Psalm 103:2–3

In his ministry on this earth, Jesus taught the kingdom of God, demonstrating its working as he healed the sick. He showed us that the kingdom is a place of healing for us if only we would trust in that fact. He often brought faith into the equation when healing the sick, and by that term he was referring to our expectancy, persistence and humility.

> As soon as they got out of the boat, people recognized Jesus. They ran throughout that whole region and carried the sick on mats to wherever they heard he was. And wherever he went—into villages, towns or countryside—they placed the sick in the market-places. They begged him to let them touch even the edge of his cloak, and all who touched him were healed.
>
> *Mark 6:54–56*

This passage is an expression of the work of the kingdom. The working of miracles, especially healing, is such an integral feature of the kingdom of God that when those experiencing some doubt asked Jesus if he really was the hoped–for Messiah, he positively clarified the matter not by referring to the wonders of his teaching but to his *works*. They were signs of the kingdom, done by the King.

> After Jesus had finished instructing his twelve disciples, he went on from there to teach and preach in the towns of Galilee.
>
> When John heard in prison what Christ was doing, he

> sent his disciples to ask him, "Are you the one who was to come, or should we expect someone else?"
>
> Jesus replied, "Go back and report to John what you hear and see: The blind receive sight, the lame walk, those who have leprosy are cured, the deaf hear, the dead are raised, and the good news is preached to the poor."
>
> *Matthew 11:1–5*

On another occasion, when people crowded around him, asking him how long he intended to keep them in suspense on the question of his kingship, Jesus' plain answer was that he had already told them but they did not believe. He affirmed that the miracles he did in the name of the Father spoke for him. And heal he most certainly did. Every sick person who came to him or who was brought to him (or even when someone else came on their behalf) was healed. Nobody was turned away. Jesus was (and is) totally reliable. He showed conclusively that the expression of the kingdom on earth at the time described in the Gospels was more than adequate to deal with all kinds of sickness and injury in all the troubled people who came to him for healing. The disciples seem to have demonstrated that, too, as they obediently carried out the ministries they were given. To believe that things are now different, that the kingdom is somehow less present today than it was in the days of Jesus' earthly ministry, is unbiblical.

The problem is never on God's side, as was so amply demonstrated by Jesus. He revealed the heart of the Father through his teaching and his kingdom work. The kingdom is indeed now very present —and not in some weaker way than in New Testament times.

God is indeed completely reliable today, as ever. Jesus offered healing to everyone; he did only what he saw the Father doing, and he and the Father are one. In all that Jesus did and taught, in his perfect relationship with the Father, we can see that they were perfectly in tune with each other.

> Do not believe me unless I do what my Father does. But if I do it, even though you do not believe me, believe the miracles, that you may know and understand that the Father is in me, and I in the Father."
>
> *John 10:37–38*

If we measure God's reliability by our own experiences of prayer, or indeed by any measure at all that is not totally Christ–centred, we will miss the truth. The only valid foundation on which to base our measurement of God's trustworthiness in healing is to study the truth of the Father's heart that is revealed perfectly in Jesus in the New Testament. His reliability is absolutely perfect.

18. Does God use suffering as a megaphone to gain our attention (and to teach us things that we do not learn when life is going well)?

Such questions commonly arise out of a search to explain any delay in our receiving healing. After all, we reason, God is good so there must be some good in our continuing suffering. We know that we have a creative God—he created the whole universe—and of course he is able and willing to make something positive out of such a time delay, but to assume from this that he is the organiser of that delay is an illogical leap too far, grossly misrepresenting the nature of God as revealed in Jesus.

Suppose a mother comes to Christ after losing her only son by suicide and after she has then experienced years of agonizing meditation on the meaning of life. It does not follow from this that God orchestrated the suicide, nor that he prolonged the mother's distress in order to bring her to the cross. It simply means that the Holy Spirit was able to work good out of something terrible.

A whole set of philosophical ideas about God's activity in our lives arises from misinterpretation of the biblical evidence. If we are allowed by God to suffer (and he must be 'allowing' it or he would have healed us by now), this must be for some grand purpose in our own lives or in the lives of those to whom we minister —so the line of argument runs.

Two basic misunderstandings are feeding in at the root of this doubt, one from the story of Job and the other emerging from a reading of Paul and others that 'suffering is good for you'. For discussion of the Job question, see Question 2, *'Am I Sick for a Reason?'* An example of Paul's positive insistence that *some* suffering has its beneficial side can be seen in Romans 5:3–5.

> Not only so, but we also rejoice in our sufferings, because we know that suffering produces perseverance; perseverance, character; and character, hope. And hope does not disappoint us, because God has poured out his love into our hearts by the Holy Spirit, whom he has given us.

It is vital to understand, though, that Paul's teaching on suffering focuses on suffering *for the sake of the gospel.* He never exalts suffering caused by illness. Such verses as those quoted above, are sometimes taken out of context or misapplied, and are often wrongly preached as meaning that being ill has its mystical benefits and that we should be satisfied with taking comfort from the fact that God loves us. He does, of course. And we are indeed to rejoice, whatever the circumstances. But he does not want us to be ill; he is our healer!

Encouragement to 'look on the bright side', and assurances that 'every cloud has a silver lining', are a long way from the liberating truth that by the Saviour's wounds you are healed. How easily doubt can pump back into people's belief systems when they entertain these two entirely false premises: that God is not wholly compassionate and is frequently unwilling to heal. Jesus is never depicted as leaving people in their sicknesses and their suffering in order (mystically) to do them good! Commendable suffering, as Paul and others refer to it, has to do with the way in which a climate of persecution is to be faced. He refers in positive terms both to the suffering in his own life from a range of personal hardships as he carries out his commission from the Lord, and to the experience of persecution in the life of the church at the hands of the Roman and Jewish authorities. And how Paul himself suffered! In 2 Corinthians 11:23–28 he reminds us that he was often close to death; eight times whipped by various authorities; he was stoned; shipwrecked three times (and once adrift at sea for a night and a day); in regular danger from floods, robbers, religious zealots and pagans. Let down by his false friends, he lived a life of hard toil; regularly endured sleepless nights and suffered hunger, thirst, inadequate clothing and shelter. These are trials or tribulations, not illnesses. Paul does not refer to any illness of his as constituting 'suffering'.

This also explains why, at the start of the Epistle of James, Christians are instructed to 'consider it pure joy' when they face trials, but are nonetheless encouraged to seek prayer for healing when they are sick (5:14–15). There is no disharmony here: the tests and trials of Chapter One of that epistle refer to persecution, not illness. God does not use sickness as a megaphone to address the sick person; his will is for the sick to be healed.

19. Does healing always have to seem instantaneous?

No, it rarely is. One of the key factors in realising healing is persistence in prayer. Much divine healing is missed at healing services and renewal meetings because we lack understanding of this. We think that when we have prayed once it is all up to God and the supplicant. There seems to us to be nothing more we can do about it. We forget that Christ has entrusted his healing ministry to us. We are expected to *keep going* until we reach the desired objective.

This idea of persistence is not to be confused with being faithful. Faithfulness is vital too, of course, but persistence is the further ingredient which is so essential in the healing ministry. It demonstrates trust. It is often tempting to receive prayer and then give up when the desired healing does not quickly arrive, but this is illogical. We would not take that approach when visiting the doctor's surgery. If our local medical practitioner were to diagnose some skin disease, for example, and then write out a prescription note for us to take to the pharmacy, we would not then throw down the note before even crossing the street when we realise that the disease has not yet left us. On the contrary, we acquire the medicine and continue with it until the required effect is achieved. If this does not happen in the expected time–frame then we are encouraged to re–visit the doctor for further treatment. In the same way, divine healing is something that, generally speaking, has to be pursued. As we press up into God so he presses down to us. He responds to persistent expectancy as he draws us to his knee. This is not to say that a demonstrable improvement in our physical condition cannot be gained within minutes. That can happen. It does mean that persistence is a vital element in our faith expectancy.

Jesus showed us the need to press onwards into healing. We recall that there was once a partial healing of a blind man, followed by further ministry to restore fully the man's vision.

> They came to Bethsaida, and some people brought a blind man and begged Jesus to touch him. He took the blind man by the hand and led him outside the village. When he had spit on the man's eyes and put his hands on him, Jesus asked, "Do you see anything?"
>
> He looked up and said, "I see people; they look like trees walking around."
>
> Once more Jesus put his hands on the man's eyes. Then his eyes were opened, his sight was restored, and he saw everything clearly.
>
> *Mark 8:22–25*

Jesus teaches us to be persistent in prayer through the parable of the persistent widow and the unjust judge (see Luke 18:1–7), and the story of the reluctant neighbour.

In the Old Testament, Naaman, the Syrian general with leprosy, who went to see Elisha for healing, was told to submerge himself in the river Jordan seven times before the disease left him. Again, both Elijah and Elisha only managed to see a young boy's life restored after very persistent ministry.

The need for us to persist in prayer is a consistent biblical theme. If we expect that divine healing should always be instantaneous then we will be led into doubt when that is not the way it happens, for we begin to think, quite wrongly, that healing might not be God's will for the person. It is always God's will, and we need to press into it.

20. Are we just tourists in the world of the miraculous?

Do we go to healing meetings to receive God's healing mercy or to pray for others, or to marvel at the miracles? Are we merely 'rubber–necking tourist' observers?

We are not called merely to watch others, but to *participate* in the work of the kingdom. We Christians must not let our lives run along in the ordinary way; our lives should bear witness that we are God's new creation, and that his power is at work in us. Tourism, in all its forms can, of course, be a fulfilling experience, broadening our outlook on life and helping us to gain a greater understanding and appreciation of the problems and aspirations of our fellow human beings in this wonderful world in which we live. We gasp in wonder, too, at God's creativity, and carry home a sense of well–being at having been there.

The apostle John, in his first letter to the believers, wrote:

> For everything in the world—the cravings of sinful man, the lust of his eyes and the boasting of what he has and does—comes not from the Father but from the world. The world and its desires pass away, but the man who does the will of God lives forever.
>
> *1 John 2:16–17*

We have to actually *do* the will of God, not just go through life like tourists, with our cravings for spiritual experiences and boasting of where we have been and what we have seen while we were there. Our existence need not be ordinary. There is something you can do that nobody else has done, and that is to bring a member of your family, a close friend or someone in your workplace into the healing presence of Jesus. Many people have been released, by the ministry of a Christian friend or a relative, from a life governed by sickness;

they have come to know Jesus Christ as their Saviour, Lord and healer, and have gone on in their turn to be active in ministry to others.

The kingdom of God is not a tourist attraction where we can just stand and gaze; it is a place for us to really live in, doing the work Jesus gave his disciples to do, in the power of the Holy Spirit. We are to go out into the world and preach the gospel, healing the sick and telling them, "The kingdom of God is near you." That is not tourism, it is discipleship.

21. I believe for others, but not so well for myself. Is this OK?

This question usually stems from a commonly held misunderstanding that a particular healing is the result of an arbitrary 'decision' by God. But we need to be aware that God's will is utterly consistent, in perfect accordance with his own self–revelation in the Scriptures. If it were not so, we would have to say that God does not always give what he promises. He is faithful to his word and his covenants. Consider this scenario: if I were to minister for healing to ten lepers, should I expect God to have a different answer for each of them? —This one to be healed; that one to remain in his sickness; another to be healed next year, perhaps? Of course not. I need only to look at how Jesus healed to know that, in the matter of healing, God's will is the same for all.

Firstly, we need to know that healing flows like a river out of heaven, a mercy–flow, released on Calvary. It should never be thought of as a question of, 'Will it come to me or them?' Rather, it is a question of our willingness to jump into that river of God's mercy. If you doubt this, jumping into that 'river of mercy' is going to mean changing your mind, as Thomas needed to do.

> Now Thomas (called Didymus), one of the Twelve, was not with the disciples when Jesus came. So the other disciples told him, "We have seen the Lord!"
>
> But he said to them, "Unless I see the nail marks in his hands and put my finger where the nails were, and put my hand into his side, I will not believe it."
>
> *John 20:24–25*

And this is so often the lot of doubters: their doubts cause them to miss out on blessings they could have enjoyed. Jesus had come back to spend time with his disciples; Thomas the doubter was not there to see it, and he did not believe their witness. But displayed here is the abundant grace and love of God: Jesus came back again a week later, and gave the doubter another opportunity to believe:

> A week later his disciples were in the house again, and Thomas was with them. Though the doors were locked, Jesus came and stood among them and said, "Peace be with you!" Then he said to Thomas, "Put your finger here; see my hands. Reach out your hand and put it into my side. Stop doubting and believe."
>
> *John 20:26–27*

Do not be like doubting Thomas a moment longer; do not miss out on any of the blessings God has in store for you. Heed the words of Jesus to Thomas: 'Stop doubting and believe.' Do not doubt that God's blessings are for you. Such doubt may stem from false humility. Know that Calvary was for *you*. The wounds of Jesus were for *your* healing, as well as for others. While it is sometimes difficult to imagine that the living God might touch us, and it may be relatively easier to believe that he will touch others, we know that, in his unconditional love, he gave Thomas another opportunity to believe; and he offers that to you. If we have faith for others and yet not for ourselves then we have not yet seen that Jesus is the embodiment of the Father's heart. Jesus healed all who came to him; his will is to heal you, too!

22. Does God still heal today? If so, then why does God not heal all sickness now? Why does God let so many youngsters die? Why do so many wonderful Christians suffer?

Yes: God certainly does heal today! Any Christ–centred ministry that consistently proclaims the good news of the kingdom of God will see it happen over and over again, to a tremendous variety of people with many different illnesses. But why not everyone? Would it not be a wonderful thing if there were no pain and no suffering in the world? It really does seem so unfair that children, and many beautiful Christians, should still go on suffering!

There are two distinct issues here and they should be kept apart to avoid confusion and doubt. First of all, the use of the word 'unfair': the very thought that being singled out and struck down is unfair is itself quite telling. At least we can clearly rule out God as being the source of sickness and injury because his unconditional and forgiving love is all–inclusive and, therefore, he cannot be unfair. He can only be the same Almighty God with love toward every one of us. We were all created in his image, and in him there is no sickness.

> Then God said, "Let us make man in our image, in our likeness, and let them rule over the fish of the sea and the birds of the air, over the livestock, over all the earth, and over all the creatures that move along the ground." So God created man in his own image, in the image of God he created him; male and female he created them.
>
> *Genesis 1:26–27*

A little later we read that, 'God saw all that he had made, and it was very good' (1:31a). There was absolutely no sickness in the Garden of Eden. That was how God intended things to be: mankind would walk in obedience and enjoy perfect health. Adam and Eve were disobedient and, as a consequence, they (and hence all their descendants) were cast out of the Garden into the world. Sickness, injury and death came into the human experience. It has been so ever since. This does not sit easily with our modern ideas about individuals and their rights, of course. But the effects of humankind's sinfulness operate like ripples spreading out from a single point. What we do affects others. The sin of Adam and Eve affects us like a disease from which every member of the human race suffers —in different ways. Some effects are indirect. Think of how environmental pollution, often caused by man's lack of love (care) for his neighbours, has blighted the lives of those who live downwind or downstream of the source. Individuals we may be, but we affect others and are affected by their actions in so many ways. In a much deeper sense, sin has affected the human race corporately. There is something in the nature of man which is proud, seeks independence of God and his perfect law of love, and which is prone to seek the best interests of self rather than others.

Secondly, the feeling that something unfair is going on

presupposes that God ignores the plight of some of his people. This idea of an uncaring and remote Deity breeds doubt (and reduces faith–expectancy) very quickly. But how do we know what God is really like? We simply need to look at Jesus, for he is the true revelation of the Father. Jesus did not account for any lack of healing (e.g. that familiar problem in his home town) by referring to a putative remote and uncaring God. No, the picture of the Father that he conveyed to us was always of a loving Father, full of love and concern for each and every one of his children. That is the image of God we must grasp, for it is the truth that Jesus constantly taught and demonstrated.

The fact that some people are not healed today has much to do with the sort of theology that begins from a sceptical position and breeds doubt and unbelief; and it is connected with a lack of real expectancy amongst the people of God. All too often, when we minister, we do not seek healing from Jesus with a child–like expectancy, persistence and humility.

The fact is that God has entrusted the work of healing the sick to the church, and has provided the power to do the work —the power that comes from him alone, from God the Holy Spirit. As we become open to the Holy Spirit, receive more from him, and minister in his power, we see more people healed. So part of the answer to the problem is to understand and move in that 'delegated' authority which is ours, as part of the commission Jesus has given to his disciples in every age. We should be asking not so much why God does not sovereignly intervene as why his church does not get on with doing more of what it has been told by him to do.

There will surely come a time when all we long for will happen. Christ will return, illness will be banished, and we shall have complete healing in body, mind and spirit. There will be a restoration of what was lost in the Garden of Eden. In the meantime, let us humbly consider the possibility of our own dereliction of duty. Could one reason for there being so much sickness around us be that we have not followed our Lord's great commission in Matthew 28:18–20?

23. Why is so much prayer apparently not answered?

There certainly seems to be much more unanswered prayer loosed off into the heavenlies today than there was two thousand years ago. It is everyone's experience that some we pray for are not healed. We have to choose between at least three possible reactions to this truth. Firstly, we can simply ignore the apparent drop in prayer 'productivity' since the days of the New Testament, and keep on hoping, as we pray for those for whom we care, when they are sick and injured. But some then start to feel that they have no real reason to suppose, if we continue praying tomorrow in the same way that we did yesterday, that anything will be any different. Secondly, some are tempted to conclude that Jesus is somehow unreliable nowadays. Those who take that tack are worshipping a different Jesus than the one who is depicted in the Gospels. Warning bells should be ringing. Thirdly, and more optimistically, we can set out to discover what we have lost and how to retrieve it!

So what *have* we lost? We have wrapped up all our past prayer 'failure' as being something to do with the mystery of it all. We either ignore past 'failure' of prayer or develop complex theology to excuse it. Either way, we have, by and large, given up all effort to grasp the simple clarity of the gospel message about the kingdom. In fact, healing and miracles are not mysterious in the way that many people think. They are not to be thought of as very exceptional divine acts bestowed in reaction to powerful praying; rather, they are, by God's grace, always available from him. The point is that we need to soak expectantly in the river of mercy that flows constantly from heaven. The New Testament repeatedly tells us that Jesus and the apostles performed miracles, including many healings. It seems to have been 'naturally' supernatural Christian living.

> "And these signs will accompany those who believe: In my name they will drive out demons; they will speak in new tongues; they will pick up snakes with their hands; and when they drink deadly poison, it will not hurt them at all; they will place their hands on sick people, and they will get well."
>
> *Mark 16:17–18*

> The apostles performed many miraculous signs and wonders among the people. And all the believers used to meet together in Solomon's Colonnade.
>
> *Acts 5:12*

In contrast, our expectancy of God to heal (of which we only need a mustard seed) is all but gone. Jesus consistently explained healing on the basis of both the minister's and the supplicant's expectancy. In the story of the healing of the woman with the issue of blood, he clearly considered her expectancy to be a major factor in the bringing about of the miracle.

> Then the woman, knowing what had happened to her, came and fell at his feet and, trembling with fear, told him the whole truth.
>
> He said to her, "Daughter, your faith has healed you. Go in peace and be freed from your suffering."
>
> *Mark 5:33–34*

With his disciples he put down to their lack of expectancy their failure to heal a boy. The New Testament explains the failure of Jesus himself to heal many in his own home town because of their unbelief in him as Saviour, healer and Lord. We lack persistence in ministry, too. We can tell from Jesus's attitude to illness that God's will is to see healing of all spiritual, psychological and physical sickness, but this does not necessarily mean that everyone gets healed immediately if they have trusting faith. Whilst some healing is immediate, there may be other times when there are other things that must first be overcome. Jesus's teaching on persistence in prayer is made abundantly clear in two parables: the story of the unjust Judge (see Luke 18:2) and the story of the man who went to his friend's house at night to ask for bread; because of the man's boldness, the bread was given. (See Luke 11:5–8). The message is that we, too, need to be both persistent and bold. Some people do not receive healing except by persistent believing prayer. Lack of persistence and boldness is part of the answer to our question. In many cultures we have also lost our humility over matters of healing. We are cynical about the reality of the things that Christ has won for us on the cross, and our minds are filled with the knowledge and memories of abuses, culturally unacceptable ministry styles and failed attempts of our own in the past. All this has to be laid down, freeing us to come, and come again, to the living Lord who heals all our diseases. We can build nothing on the mixed experience of the church down the centuries since Jesus' ministry on earth. We can only build reliably on Jesus Christ. He revealed that the will of the Father is for everyone to be healed. He revealed this over and over again, by healing everyone in the crowds that flocked to him. He revealed this unwaveringly, by never turning anyone away unhealed.

24. Could God be delaying his healing?

We have prayed, we have fasted, and as yet nothing is happening. Could God be delaying his healing in order to bring about some greater purpose out of the circumstances? Even worse, in such situations it is often claimed that God has revealed through intercessory prayer that healing will not be given, and that those who are praying are to let go of the supplicant in their hearts. On the other hand, we can often feel that God delays his healing for such a long time that our friend or relative dies before God can get to them. Sometimes we ask ourselves about hidden sins in the sick person's life which God would want to deal with first, and at other times we surmise that the supplicant may not really want to be healed at all. None of this is of God, it is simply and only an outworking of the intercessor's doubt about Jesus as healer. No, this is not the nature of God as revealed through Jesus. Jesus is our only true revelation of God, and nowhere in the Gospels does he ever turn away a sick person for some indeterminate period of time to await some greater and as yet undefined work of God. He healed everyone who asked him and, by inference, very quickly. He even healed the man with a withered hand on the Sabbath, thus demonstrating to us that healing will not even wait for one day. So why is there sometimes a delay? Two things are usually needed for healing to take place. We have to create a faith environment around the supplicant (a state of expectancy through the teaching of the good news of Jesus). Then we ourselves must pray in faith (expectancy). We should not forget that we cannot see perfectly into the heart of the supplicant, and there may be some degree of doubt and double–minded thinking going on. Only when we approach the throne of grace with simple, uncluttered and child–like simplicity can we expect to see the kingdom of heaven unfold before our eyes.

It may be fruitful, therefore, to pray the Holy Spirit for revelation about such things as double–minded doubt. The word 'double–minded' does not describe something we would ordinarily think of as evil, it simply means the holding of an alternative view. On the one hand the Gospels prove the will of God to be healing, uninterrupted and generous beyond describing. On the other hand, we humans can accept God's love and then raise up all sorts of 'Ah, but...' questions and statements. These are all 'doubt' and we should not really expect to receive when we are in this sort of double–minded state:

> If any of you lacks wisdom, he should ask God, who gives generously to all without finding fault, and it will be given to him. But when he asks, he must believe and not doubt, because he who doubts is like a wave of the sea, blown and tossed by the wind. That man should not think he will receive anything from the Lord; he is a double-minded man, unstable in all he does.
>
> *James 1:5–8*

Such double–mindedness is usually the only block to the flow of God's healing grace. We need no condemnation here, but gentle and compassionate exploration of our own spirit's expectancy of God. When that exploration is happily and successfully exhausted, we may prayerfully approach the supplicant, praying all the while for grace in our attempts to help them.

25. Does God heal minds as well as bodies? Is the healing of the mind more or less difficult than the healing of the body?

The healing of the mind can be split into three categories for the purposes of understanding ministry. Firstly there is ministry to mental illness which covers a wide range of dysfunction —from mild mood swings right up to life–threatening and life–destroying illnesses. At the one end of the range these things seem of little importance and at the other end, for the medically uneducated, these things seem completely mysterious and virtually unapproachable.

As with any form of physical illness, a major barrier to receiving healing is not our lack of comprehension of an illness in itself but the wholly understandable, scientific view that some things are more difficult to heal than others. As this is so in the medical world, we mistakenly think it must be true in the kingdom of God. But there is no biblical evidence to support this idea. Jesus did not find 'serious' diseases any more difficult than what we might describe today as relatively inconsequential ones —he healed them all. There surely would have been those suffering from mental illness in the crowds that surrounded the Lord.

Until recently in church history, mental illness has been classified in the Christian mind as being something demonic. Thanks to present–day advances in medical science and the treatment of such illnesses, we now know very differently; the incidence of demonic involvement in mental illness is probably no greater than in physical disease. In fact, just as with any other form of serious illness, we need to overcome doubt if we are to see consistent healing taking place.

Secondly, the mind can be said to be 'not whole' to the degree with which we lead our lives out of kilter with God. This may, of course, be the result of wilful and deliberate sin but often stems from all sorts of other reasons, much to do with the changing role of the church in society and how that is perceived by the public at large. For the individual, deepening of the life with God, which is an important factor in the restoration of mental health, is only a function of prayer, of spending time with him, learning to hear and respond to the voice of Jesus. Jesus spoke of our relationship by comparing it to sheep following their master. The sheep, "...follow him because they know his voice." (See John 10:3–5). Part of healing ministry is helping people to come to a place where they can begin to hear that voice.

Thirdly, we need to consider the damage done to our present ability to relate to God and to other people by the wounds of the past. Not one of us has had perfect parents, perfect teachers and perfect playmates in youth; we are all scarred in some way or other. Most of the bad ways in which we react to those around us are actually sins reacting off past hurts. Such moments in time may be lovingly redeemed by God through prayer and ministry. Peter had denied his Lord three times by a fire and afterwards was not even counted among the disciples. In the simple act of lighting another fire and asking Peter three times to re–affirm his love, the worst moment in Peter's life is redeemed and his life and ministry is completely restored. (See John 21:9–18). This is a message of repentance and forgiveness; it is also a message about the restoration of interior peace which Peter needed so much.

In all respects, the healing of the mind is as much a part of the healing ministry as is the healing of our bodies. God desires wholeness for us in every way.

26. Whose fault is it that I am not healed after prayer? Is it me or the minister or God?

This raises a serious pastoral issue. Many who are prayed for and do not receive healing move into feelings of being rejected by God and, as we are all steeped in the blame game, we look for scapegoats. This is our human way of lashing out in order to avenge our rejection. However, if progress is to be made, we would all be much better off seeking the healer rather than spend that spiritual energy looking around for someone to take the blame.

We need three things to receive healing: expectancy, persistence and humility. Firstly, we will fall away from the needed humility straight away if we are blaming anyone, the minister or oneself, for failure, rather than going on seeking Jesus. Secondly, much receiving of healing is missed simply because we try once and give up if results are not immediate and sustained. The reason for the scarcity of persistence in the church is usually a lack of understanding that it is necessary at all, and a lack of faith that it will do any good to press on. We fear that we may be raising hopes unfairly, or putting the supplicant's faith at risk, and yet Jesus himself taught us through two parables that persistence is essential. Thirdly, there are doubts. We may have difficulties, both consciously and subconsciously, in fully and simply accepting Jesus as healer. These doubts are the things that prevent the receiving of healing and should be approached, discussed and overcome in honest and Bible based ways. A minister's fear that supplicants (or even they themselves) may lose faith allows room for just enough doubt (that God will act consistently and reliably) to prevent them from receiving healing. It also prevents many leaders from humbly admitting that they failed to fulfil what they suspect, in theory, they should have been able to do, and from having their beliefs and attitudes adjusted by God. Instead, many ministers justify themselves and the supplicant as having no faults in the arena of healing, at the expense of God's reputation for being compassionate and completely reliable. This regrettable theology creates serious pastoral issues for future healing situations, for those who hear their justifications. Blame arises if the person wanting healing comes to the minister much as we would approach a doctor's surgery, or a superstore in search of what we would like to buy. If our needs are not immediately fulfilled, we complain. A healthier picture, without any potential for blaming, is to see that we Christians are all part of the body of Christ, humbly striving to find answers together about our relationship with God and our ability to receive what is already given.

Expectancy, persistence and humility may be lacking in some way in the supplicant but they may also be wanting in the minister, and in the surrounding congregation if there is one. No–one is to blame; we only have shortfalls in our understanding to overcome together.

Christ wills that all supplicants should receive healing, whether or not the minister is able to accomplish that completely with them.

27. If I get ill again, can I be healed more than once?

Of course this is very possible. Nowhere did Jesus check any supplicant's past medical history before healing a sickness. He did not withhold his mercy on the grounds that someone had been ill before. And Jesus is the true revelation of the Father's heart.

There must have been many in the multitudes who were going back for a second shot at being healed, not because the first attempt had failed but because the sickness had re–appeared. Jesus did not discriminate; he healed them all. This should not surprise us. If we catch a cold one winter and are healed by a combination of our in–built healing resources and prayer, we may still catch another cold next winter! The fact that a particular sickness can happen more than once in our lives is not some fault in the one who prayed, nor in the process of divine healing. To be sick we need to be presented with two separate things: a weakness and a trigger. Weakness plus trigger equals illness. Particular weakness may be inherited (our scientists are discovering this more and more) or it may be present in our bodies through injury, the leading of stressful lifestyles and so on. Triggers are such things as germs, seeds, head–on collisions with harder objects, insufficient sleep, etc. The range of weaknesses is too vast to be easily discernible, and the range of triggers is endless. Our susceptibility to all these things is probably the result of the Fall of man into sin, sickness and death.

Into this mess flows the river of God's healing power, released at the moment of Jesus' death and, because he now lives and reigns in heaven, continuing to flow without ceasing. The river knows no limits. It makes no judgements and has no conditions. It simply flows. It is wonderful if we can discern the original weakness and see that healed. If this can happen, then in–coming triggers would simply have no effect since, as we have said, both trigger and weakness need to be present. However, our medical and scientific professions have not developed this way, preferring by and large to approach from the angle of cure after the event. This is hardly surprising; facing such subjects as stress and sinful lifestyles demands too many questions of us.

So we cut and carve our bodies and alter their chemical balances with drugs; in this way, vast amounts of suffering have been relieved, but sickness recurs. This earthly approach does not dam up the river. God's mercy flow never ceases—it never even pauses for breath, so to speak!

If illness re–emerges, we retreat to the river bank again,

giving glory to the God who loves us, and there he heals us once more.

For further reading see No. 46 *Does this sort of healing last?*

28. Can I intercede by suffering for others?

It is sometimes believed by devout intercessors that we might somehow be able to reduce the level of pain and sickness in those we love and pray for by drawing that sickness into ourselves.

There is, no doubt, some sacrificial component to loving another person, which is coming into play here. Watching a child or a lifelong partner racked with pain or crippled with disfigurement raises up all sorts of emotions, and a servant heart that longs to carry the burden for the sufferer. If somehow we could handle the disease for them then, we think, they might not have to be so oppressed by it. We imagine that if only we could take the sickness and pain upon ourselves then our loved ones would not need to suffer any more. These are not merely true human emotions, they also reflect an intrinsic part of the work of the cross. If we sense such feelings within us then we may well be in touch with the deep cries of the Spirit of Christ living within us. However, it is a very wrong thing that we should attempt to take the dis-ease of others into ourselves, because in so doing we deny a large part of the work on the cross and withhold ourselves from its power. The sting of sickness, tragedy and death has already been drawn. The work of the cross is complete. We must never forget that the oppression of all our griefs, sorrows, pains and sicknesses has already been laid on Jesus. Here is Isaiah's prophetic promise on this subject.

> He was despised and rejected by men,
> a man of sorrows, and familiar with suffering.

Like one from whom men hide their faces
he was despised, and we esteemed him not.
Surely he took up our infirmities
and carried our sorrows,
yet we considered him stricken by God,
smitten by him, and afflicted.
But he was pierced for our transgressions,
he was crushed for our iniquities;
the punishment that brought us peace was upon him,
and by his wounds we are healed.
We all, like sheep, have gone astray,
each of us has turned to his own way;
and the LORD has laid on him the iniquity of us all.

Isaiah 53:3–6

Jesus was the ultimate and complete sacrifice for us.

Just as there were many who were appalled at him
—his appearance was so disfigured
beyond that of any man
and his form marred beyond human likeness–

Isaiah 52:14

This was all done for us in his crucifixion so that we might enable our loved ones to press their troubles into the foot of Calvary's cross. To pull the difficulties of others into ourselves, so that *we* can be that sacrifice for them, may even be described as being occult, as it denies and actively avoids the victorious work of the King on Calvary.

In adverse family conditions we would do better to heed this storm narrative, recounted in Luke 8:22–25.

One day Jesus said to his disciples, "Let's go over to the other side of the lake." So they got into a boat and set out.

As they sailed, he fell asleep. A squall came down on the lake, so that the boat was being swamped, and they were in great danger. The disciples went and woke him, saying, "Master, Master, we're going to drown!" He got up and rebuked the wind and the raging waters; the storm subsided, and all was calm.

"Where is your faith?" he asked his disciples.

In fear and amazement they asked one another, "Who is this? He commands even the winds and the water, and they obey him."

Luke 8:22–25

When our friends and loved ones are in danger from the storms of life, we should expectantly go to the Lord who commands even the winds and the water, and they obey him.

29. Is not death a great healer?

Will we be better off where we are going? Death is often described as a 'blessed release', especially when the deceased has been very ill for a long time, with little or no quality of life. Sometimes, out of love and concern for the sufferer, we even pray for this release, but we had better pray at the same time for God's mercy to be upon their souls while they are still living. Of course, the result of Christian death is that we shall receive what is, in a sense, the fullest healing of all: a new, resurrection body; so the general assertion that death is healing must depend on what is going to happen to us afterwards. We will all have to face our God and account for our lives.

"At that time Michael, the great prince who protects your people, will arise. There will be a time of distress

> such as has not happened from the beginning of nations until then. But at that time your people—everyone whose name is found written in the book—will be delivered. Multitudes who sleep in the dust of the earth will awake: some to everlasting life, others to shame and everlasting contempt."
>
> *Daniel 12:1–2*

For the redeemed there is a sure hope, for Jesus said:

> "I tell you the truth, he who believes has everlasting life. I am the bread of life."
>
> *John 6:47–48*

The bland assertion that death is a sort of healing does, however, serve to give us a comfortable sense of absolution from any responsibilities in the matter. We are the bearers of the healing word of God. From a kingdom viewpoint, sickness and injury are like a thief who comes only to steal and kill and destroy; Jesus has come so that we may have life, and have it to the full. We have two options here. We can take the risk of praying that a friend or relative should pass out of this life, a risk if we are not quite certain of their likely destination. On the other hand, we know that our healing King has come to offer us salvation, including healing from injury and sickness, and that we can step into that healing kingdom during this life on earth. There must surely have been many dying people who came to Jesus in the multitude and were healed. There were certainly many in severe pain and Jesus healed them all.

For further reading, see No. 31 *Do we have to get ill to die?*

30. Why does healing seem to happen more in places like Africa?

One of the most common doubts that is considered but rarely spoken is this: do some cultural variations around the world make it easier for some people groups to receive healing? If so, then those of us who live in Western (so-called) civilisation need not consider healing, because we must be, for some reason or another, excluded. 'It would not work here anyway,' so this line of thinking runs. 'Is it not only in Africa that signs and wonders prosper? Is it only where people become over–excited that they believe things happen to them?'

There are three major flaws with such assumptions. Firstly, there are many African countries where healing miracles abound and many where few are recorded. The outflowing of God's grace is not an exclusively African thing. Secondly, there are many other places around the world, North and South America, the Far East, and so on, where healing miracles abound. Thirdly, Europe is far from being bereft of such graces — there abound numerous centres for healing that are mightily blessed. Away from the glare of public attention, God's healing blessings are experienced all over the globe. Healing takes place throughout all varieties of different denominations, too. It can happen through anyone —sometimes just the ministers, and sometimes none of them. It happens during different services, eucharistic or otherwise. The keys to release the receiving of healing are not culturally or nationally based at all; it is simply easier for some people to assimilate them than it is for others. The three major keys are expectancy, persistence and humility before God. Our ethnic background is not one of the issues. The greatest block to healing is not race but doubt: questioning, excusing, avoiding, cynical doubt. It is easy to see that, as a broad generalisation, some nations may find simple and uncluttered expectancy easier than others.

The atmosphere in the kingdom of God is one of restoration —most of our wrong beliefs about healing have arisen simply because we have never been taught the subject in an informed manner. How can every nation see the kingdom restoring its members?

> He called a little child and had him stand among them. And he said: "I tell you the truth, unless you change and become like little children, you will never enter the kingdom of heaven."
>
> *Matthew 18:2–3*

Healing is a supernatural result of our response to Jesus and, as such, can be received by any member of any faith, and even by those who have no religion with which they readily identify themselves. It is often those Christians who have a 'sophisticated' spirituality and complex theologies and philosophies who have the greater difficulty in receiving healing because of them. Those with a more child–like approach often receive more readily, while other children of God miss out. After Jesus had finished his first sermon, he tried to explain this difficulty to his listeners.

> "I tell you the truth," he continued, "no prophet is accepted in his hometown. I assure you that there were many widows in Israel in Elijah's time, when the sky was shut for three and a half years and there was a severe famine throughout the land. Yet Elijah was not sent to any of them, but to a widow in Zarephath in the region of Sidon. And there were many in Israel with leprosy in the time of Elisha the prophet, yet not one of them was cleansed —only Naaman the Syrian."
>
> All the people in the synagogue were furious when they heard this. They got up, drove him out of the town,

and took him to the brow of the hill on which the town was built, in order to throw him down the cliff. But he walked right through the crowd and went on his way.

Luke 4:24–30

Jesus is telling them that outsiders often receive healing more easily than the local inhabitants. He is pointing to those on the margins, showing us that God draws us there to minister when the children of God so often miss out on the blessings. In both the Old Testament stories he refers to we find great expectancy, persistence and humility. The two prophets mentioned by Jesus were used to heal foreigners because they possessed those keys which are so often lacking —expectancy, persistence and humility before God. In any part of the world, where those keys are present, we see kingdom works taking place.

31. Do we have to get ill to die?

We can receive healing throughout our lives without having to die from an illness. Sickness is not a prerequisite for death. There are a number of examples of this illness–free dying found both in Scripture and in the everyday experience of Christian life. Even though some of us do die through sickness, there is no condemnation —on the contrary, we are made whole in our dying.

Smith Wigglesworth is an example of someone who died without being sick or injured. It is said that he did not even have any tooth decay. Even elderly people who are generally healthy do die without any apparent sickness being the cause of their leaving us. The idea that pre–death sickness in our old age is fairly well inevitable, that it is somehow a method that God often uses to bring us to the point of dying, creates serious doubt for the very ill, and for those who love them. Healing is possible, and is God's will, right up to the point of our death. This view is quite consistent with the Father's will as it has been revealed to us through Jesus. There would certainly have been elderly and dying people in those multitudes who came to him, and he healed them all. Such 'doubting doctrines' as the inevitability of sickness in old age are responsible for many untimely deaths by injury and sickness. Persuading people not to ask for healing, or perhaps to ask in a double–minded fashion, reflects doubt concerning God's purposes, and it is that doubt which is harmful. The sick person is hindered from coming to Jesus in simple faith. Doubting doctrines have made it all so complex and mysterious for us. We might ask our doctors the question, 'Do some of us die of things that are medically inexplicable?' Many medical authorities often believe, as an axiom, that there must be a specific cause of death. They then set out to justify this standpoint by finding and naming one even when none is obvious. However, there are quite a number of deaths worldwide that are attributed to 'sudden death syndrome', because there is no medical explanation found for that person's dying.

The expression 'natural causes' on a death certificate can mean that there was no discernible reason found for death, even after a post mortem. To add to this, there are numbers of apparently healthy people who die instantly, or at any rate almost instantly, in battle or in traffic accidents, of heart attacks, strokes, accidents at work or in the home, murder and other kinds of trauma massive enough to kill them. There have also been many martyrs down the centuries who experienced massive and life–threatening injury only moments before death. Some of our medical scientists might argue here that there was an overwhelming lack of health in all these situations, but it is possible that all of them felt in perfect health one moment and found themselves in heaven in the next.

So we do not have to be sick in order to die; death by sickness is certainly not inevitable. Healing prayer should go on being a working resource for us until we need it no longer —either because we have died or because we are completely well. Until our death, healing is always available to us through trust and expectancy in Jesus Christ. James chapter five makes no artificial distinction at all between certain people who are supposed to die and those who are meant to live. On the contrary, the implication is that all believers can receive the wonders of believing, healing prayer all the days of their life. We should pray the prayer of faith over the sick, however old or ill they may be, and we should expect them to be healed.

32. How should we pray for healing?

Consider two ways in which God works in his kingdom to bring healing and miracles into the lives of his children. Firstly, he uses our intercession. This we may describe as Route A. We, like the four friends lowering the paralysed man down through the roof, bring the supplicant to the feet of Jesus and submit our requests on their behalf. So it is that we are exhorted: 'Pray in the Spirit on all occasions with all kinds of prayers and requests. With this in mind, be alert and always keep on praying for all the saints' (Ephesians 6:18). Intercession for healing had been commended in the Old Testament, too:

> Then the king said to the man of God, "Intercede with the LORD your God and pray for me that my hand may be restored." So the man of God interceded with the LORD, and the king's hand was restored and became as it was before.
>
> *1 Kings 13:6*

Route A is the only one available to us when the supplicant lives at a distance or would not, for whatever reason, be open to receiving direct ministry. Some such prayers of intercession are answered in the way we request, but many are not, the reasons for the latter lying either in the mystery of God or in the church's lack of understanding about their role in the kingdom. One problem with Route A is obvious —those who would minister to the sick find it harder to help them to be open to the work of Jesus and to receive what is already given. Since the incarnation of our Lord Jesus Christ, Route B is the preferred route, and its basis is this:

> His intent was that now, through the church, the manifold wisdom of God should be made known to the rulers and authorities in the heavenly realms, according to his eternal purpose which he accomplished in Christ Jesus our Lord. In him and through faith in him we may approach God with freedom and confidence.
>
> *Ephesians 3:10–12*

The preferred route is that the church should minister God's merciful healing to the people, understanding how to express the kingdom among the people in such a way that the sick are healed —not just once in a while, but regularly and continuously. Importantly, this does not mean that we should stand with the supplicant and revert to Route A —the more popular intercession method in the presence of the supplicant — we may as well leave prayer to our quiet times and intercede for the sick at home if that is the route we are to adopt. Route B, first and foremost, involves the teaching or preaching of the kingdom and the way the kingdom works. It teaches about the King and about his ministry on earth, and how that totally reliable ministry is the only true revelation of the Father's heart. Because Jesus Christ on earth healed everyone who asked, Route B teaches that God's heart is to heal everyone who comes to him. The Father cannot move in an opposite direction to the Son.

> ...but because Jesus lives forever, he has a permanent priesthood. Therefore he is able to save completely those who come to God through him, because he always lives to intercede for them.
>
> *Hebrews 7:24–25*

Jesus taught the kingdom in this way, and he himself became, as it were, the open 'sluice gate' for the healing mercy–flow between the kingdom and this world. The apostles, too, would have taught the kingdom in this powerful way, and most around them were healed. The divine mercy to heal flowed through them as if they, too, were sluice gates. This is still the role of the church today. Now if, in him, and through faith in him, we may approach God with freedom and confidence, then what would our reaction to standing before him truly be? We would probably not stand there asking questions; we would have little option but to simply worship him. So, standing with the supplicant in the kingdom, waiting for Jesus to intercede for us, our praying becomes pure worship. The essence or heart of effective healing prayer does not consist in asking God for something we need for ourselves or for the person to whom we are trying to minister, though it will include or can lead into asking, commanding, rebuking the disorder, speaking to the condition and so on, at times, as the Spirit leads. Jesus does teach us to ask, of course, and we should not stop doing so. The point is that all those other modes of prayer activity must be based on a kind of prayer that is much deeper, more foundational: the everyday opening of our hearts to God, being with him and living with him in endless spiritual communion, and this is made possible by his grace, which we experienced when we first received Jesus and were born again by the

Spirit of God. At root, healing ministry prayer should be a constant abandonment to God, dwelling in awareness of his presence. There has to be a real desire to be in the presence of God himself, the only Giver of abundant life—forever. This is vital both for our own discipleship and to see the floodgates of healing blessing released for others. The true spirit of prayer comes in living a life of fellowship with Jesus, abiding in him.

For more on the subject see No. 16 *Should we really expect it to happen?*

Part Four

More Biblical Issues

33. What about the healing at the pool at Bethesda?

This passage from John's Gospel is often quoted when the question is asked, 'Why doesn't God heal everybody?' It appears, unusually, that Jesus picked out just one individual from a crowd of sick people around a pool, healed that person and then walked away, leaving us with the impression that the others would not be healed at that time. It looks at first glance as though Jesus selects only some to be healed. This appears to be one of those rare examples where someone did not come to Jesus for healing (or another did not come on their behalf) and yet Christ specifically seems to have sought them out in order to give them this particular gift. There are only a very few examples of such unsolicited intervention among the thousands of healings and miracles during Jesus' ministry. Another incident that comes to mind is the bringing back from death of the widow's son (Luke 7:11–18). In that account, it appears that Christ has again, as at the pool at Bethesda, surprised everyone with the miracle.

By virtue of their rarity, unsolicited healings are extraordinary, and our theology of healing ought to acknowledge that they are so. It does seem wise, cautious and practical, however, that our theological foundation for healing is based on Jesus' usual methods rather than the extraordinary occurrences where, often, a special teaching point is being made. Later on (after the healing miracle at the pool) Jesus explains that he only does what he sees the Father doing. Some seize on that statement and link it to the undeniable fact that only one person was healed at that time and place. The rare, unusual incident is mistakenly taken as showing that the Father does not wish to heal everyone.

> Some time later, Jesus went up to Jerusalem for a feast of the Jews. Now there is in Jerusalem near the Sheep Gate a pool, which in Aramaic is called Bethesda and which is surrounded by five covered colonnades. Here a great number of disabled people used to lie—the blind, the lame, the paralysed.
>
> One who was there had been an invalid for thirty-eight years. When Jesus saw him lying there and learned that he had been in this condition for a long time, he asked him, "Do you want to get well?"
>
> "Sir," the invalid replied, "I have no one to help me into the pool when the water is stirred. While I am trying to get in, someone else goes down ahead of me."
>
> Then Jesus said to him, "Get up! Pick up your mat and walk."
>
> *John 5:1–8*

Jesus asked him whether he wanted to get well. He is beginning to set up a faith environment here —implying that responding to himself and to the good news of the gospel is, in fact, the faith response that is needed; the question seems to imply that this sufferer could indeed begin to have a real hope. We always need to set up a faith environment in which healing can work. There is no evidence to suggest that anyone else around that pool had, or was prepared to have, a faith response toward Jesus. The system they were all using, the technique that the invalid was drawn away from by Jesus, was not Christ–centred but seems to have been structured on what we might think of today as superstitious beliefs —which may have allowed some degree of expectancy, but that needed to be healthily re–directed toward Jesus, rather than toward a ritual. At the Bethesda pool, the belief was that the first one in the pool when the water was troubled by an angel would be healed. This was the limit of the expectancy in that place. The results would have been very limited, too, but enough for them to have thought the procedure worth trying —enough to give the place a certain reputation. In modern times we may still have superstitious beliefs. For example, some think that God will perform miracles only in some special location, or when some especially gifted speaker is at work. This does not mean that the place or the speaker are necessarily thought of as having particular powers, just that we restrict the ministry by limiting our expectancy. Does the explanation by Jesus that he only did what he saw his Father doing mean that our Father does not want to heal everyone? That would be an inaccurate and misleading interpretation. The questions directed at Jesus, to which this answer about his unity in working with the Father was given, were not about how many he had healed but about why he had done the miracle on the Sabbath.

> For this reason the Jews tried all the harder to kill him; not only was he breaking the Sabbath, but he was even calling God his own Father, making himself equal with God.
>
> *John 5:18*

In the Bible, we are shown that God is faithful, reliable and consistent. Jesus made it clear that we need to *expect* healing; we will find that God does what he has promised.

34. Is healing in the atonement?

The issue is this: are we to think of the healing work of God as having been *completed* on the cross (i.e. in the atonement) so that it needs only to be appropriated? Two slightly different approaches are sometimes proposed instead:

1. The crucifixion is seen as being akin to the opening of a door, making healing a possibility, *through* the cross. But this is not the same as appropriating a finished work.
2. The cross was simply a guilt offering, an atonement for sin, and healing will only be fully available when Jesus returns.

So this is the debate: is divine healing in or through the atonement, or is it, to all intents and purposes, independent of the atonement? Is the work of healing finished (but yet to be fully manifested), or is it that the way of intercessory prayer has been opened for us?

If healing is part of the finished work on the cross, then we can always be certain that God will heal when we come to Christ as healer with expectancy. If, however, healing may or may not come, because the cross simply allows us prayerful access to the throne of grace, then healing must only be some sort of additional extra that is given to us when God sovereignly decides to give it. It would be as though the cross only opened a door for God to use if he wishes to. It would follow that it would be difficult to be certain, if healing is only through the atonement (as distinct from being an intrinsic part of it), that God would heal.

Consistent, personal expectancy for healing (such as Jesus enjoins as he commends faith) would be a most difficult thing to attain if this interpretation were correct, and it is not enough just to accept that God *can* do healing. We must believe that God's active will is for us to be healed. This expectancy (faith), which we can understand from Jesus' comments on so many occasions to be a major factor in healing, would, for the one who believes that healing is only through the atonement and not in it, seem to be based on something less than reliable. It would probably require a personal revelation, if not some sort of actual proof, that God wanted the person to be well, to inspire expectancy for healing. Otherwise, doubt would always be present and that could easily prevent receiving. Some, indeed, do think that a word of knowledge, or some such, is a vital prerequisite to their receiving. On the other hand, if healing is an intrinsic element of the work of Jesus on the cross, then a believer can always be certain that God wishes them to receive it, without further special revelation. The price would already have been paid, and healing would be received in the same uncluttered way that salvation is so readily taken on board.

Two of the apostles who walked with Jesus, Peter and Matthew, quite clearly connect healing with the atonement. Isaiah 53 includes verses which clearly concern healing, along with others concerning the atonement for sin. At face value, two apostolic witnesses combined with Isaiah's prophetic description of the atonement should really be enough to convince us that healing is *in* (rather than only *through*) the atonement. There is no biblical evidence to suggest that healing is not in the atonement. Some theologians offer the absence of a discussion of healing from the writings of the apostle Paul to be a biblical argument that healing must be less present in the atonement —that, although healing might be in the atonement, it would be a much lesser and much weaker benefit of the cross. At best this is a weak standpoint, as nowhere in his writings does the apostle Paul imply that healing is not in the atonement, nor even that it is a weakened part of it. In all this, it is vital to recall, of course, that there is no biblical evidence that Jesus taught healing as a subject. He, and the apostles after him, taught about the kingdom of God, and those listening were healed.

So there are three places in the Bible that clearly connect

healing with atonement, the finished work of the cross. Two of these references consist of primary apostolic witness and teaching. The third is from a primary messianic prophetic passage which is, on a number of occasions, quoted about Jesus in the New Testament. We have to balance Paul's silence on the subject against this double apostolic and prophetic witness. Jesus himself ties healing into salvation eighteen times in the Gospels by using the form of the Greek word for salvation (sozo) in situations where someone is receiving healing ministry.

Matthew quotes from Isaiah Chapter 53, and links it with healing, in a passage which is widely accepted as being a description of what Christ would accomplish at the cross:

> When evening came, many who were demon–possessed were brought to him (Jesus), and he drove out the spirits with a word and healed all the sick. This was to fulfil what was spoken through the prophet Isaiah:
>
> "He took up our infirmities
> and carried our diseases."
>
> *Matthew 8:16–17*

Matthew obviously believed that Isaiah's prophecy was being fulfilled in Christ's healing ministry, and that the prophet Isaiah was describing physical healing rather than the spiritual kind. Some argue that Matthew is not tying healing directly to the cross at this point, but he would surely have known that the Isaiah piece he quotes most certainly does! The second apostolic witness quoted is 1 Peter 2:24,

> He himself bore our sins in his body on the tree, so that we might die to sins and live for righteousness; by his wounds you have been healed.

Peter is connecting the atoning work of the cross very closely to healing and, to underline this, he quotes from Isaiah's prophecy, which itself links healing with the atonement for sin. We can then conclude quite simply that both Matthew and Peter believed that healing was in the atonement.

A short study of the passage in question, Isaiah Chapter 53, should also help us. The language and structure of this chapter does not lend support to the idea that Isaiah might have been trying to separate the work of the suffering servant from the work of healing, an important point in considering whether healing is in or through that atoning work of the cross. Only this one single Isaiah phrase separates the two apostolic quotes about healing: 'But he was pierced for our transgressions, he was crushed for our iniquities' (Isaiah 53:5a). This portion of the verse is unmistakably about the atonement; Matthew's quotation is drawn from just before it and Peter's immediately after. The Isaiah passage is not separating healing from atonement for sin, but is mixing the two things together as one. At the end of the passage in question, immediately after Peter's quote about healing, we find these words from the prophet,

> We all, like sheep, have gone astray,
> each of us has turned to his own way;
> and the LORD has laid on him
> the iniquity of us all.
>
> *Isaiah 53:6*

So this is how this part of the Isaiah passage is constructed —every alternate statement in these verses is either about healing or atonement for the forgiveness of sin. The 'took/ carried away sickness' phrase used by Matthew is followed by the 'pierced/transgression' phrase. This in turn is followed by the 'wounds/healed' phrase used by Peter, and the section is completed by the 'iniquity/on him' phrase. Isaiah is mixing together the two ideas of the Suffering Servant doing what has to be done to provide healing with his paying the price for the forgiveness of our sin and iniquity. The proposition that healing is not in the atonement overlooks the linguistic facts and structures of this passage, which does not separate the two ideas of healing provided by God and reconciliation with him. Theology often can, however, separate healing and forgiveness in the atonement without biblical license, and thereby serve to bring yet more doubt into the church on the question of the healing of the sick. An attitude of simple acceptance of healing being in the atonement — a child–like attitude — makes it much easier for us to reliably and consistently receive healing.

35. Do we have a covenant right to be healed?

If we confess our sins we are forgiven. We can confidently claim that as a truth. Some theologians ask, concerning healing: If we claim it as a covenant right, do we get it? It is sometimes said of those who believe that healing is in the atonement that they are saying just this: claim it and, if you do so with enough faith, then it is yours. It would then follow that any lack of healing is blamed on the supplicant's lack of faith.

This arrow falls wide of the mark. We do not receive forgiveness for our sins because we claim that forgiveness as a covenant right; we receive it because we kneel with contrite and repentant hearts before God. It is the cross that has made this possible. In the same way, no one receives healing because they claim it as a right. They receive it by approaching the throne of grace with expectancy, persistence and humility. Just as the floodgates of heaven's forgiveness are opened when we come to Jesus with repentant hearts, so are the floodgates of healing mercy opened by the Lord as we come to him in simple and child–like expectancy.

> When they came to the crowd, a man approached Jesus and knelt before him.
>
> "Lord, have mercy on my son," he said. "He has seizures and is suffering greatly. He often falls into the fire or into the water. I brought him to your disciples, but they could not heal him."
>
> "O unbelieving and perverse generation," Jesus replied, "how long shall I stay with you? How long shall I put up with you? Bring the boy here to me."
>
> Jesus rebuked the demon, and it came out of the boy, and he was healed from that moment. Then the disciples came to Jesus in private and asked, "Why couldn't we drive it out?"
>
> He replied, "Because you have so little faith. I tell you the truth, if you have faith as small as a mustard seed, you can say to this mountain, 'Move from here to there' and it will move. Nothing will be impossible for you."
>
> *Matthew 17:14*

God does not *choose* who or who not to heal in some mysterious way; rather, where there is the faith–expectancy, persistence and humility of which Jesus taught, he releases healing. The cross does not give us rights, but it guarantees us privileges.

36. Is it always the devil who wants us to be ill?

In terms of spiritual warfare, and Christian healing must be part of that, it is important to understand Satan's role in sickness. To understand his strategy is to avoid being misled and thereby missing out on healing miracles. Not only that, but accusations about unrepented sin can lead only to added pain and turmoil within the family of the sick person.

It is too simplistic for us to believe that, because all good things come from God, all bad things must come from Satan. Not all sicknesses, by any means, are due to the personal sin of the sufferer or the direct intervention of the devil. The fallenness of the world, for example, is also a cause of sickness. Many of our sicknesses are, we might say, quite 'neutral' in their origin (i.e. they involve neither direct personal culpability on the part of the sufferer nor directly demonic attack). We must also resist the notion that sickness is some evil in the air that is waiting only for a crack in our spiritual armour to get in. This view implies that there must be a demonic power controlling and directing the ingress and flow of all sickness. In fact, only about a quarter of the healing miracles in Jesus' ministry seem to be related in some way to demonic activity. Even under that measure we are only allowing for the specific and individual miracles mentioned in the Gospels —we do not know what proportion of sicknesses involving demonic activity was uncovered by Jesus whenever he healed a multitude of people. Simply considering Jesus's ministry, we may deduce that not all sickness is caused by evil spirits.

Modern scientific research is increasingly revealing that a large proportion of sickness comes about because of the coming together of two important factors: we have to have a weakness in the make-up of the mind or the body, and we have to have a trigger. We are discovering that more and more of our weaknesses are actually inherited through 'faulty' DNA. (The latter, like many causal factors, could be regarded as part of the general effect of the Fall, as God's original creation was perfect and we can assume that the DNA with which Adam and Eve were created would have been flawless.) The trigger could be anything from a germ to stress, or to otherwise normal changes within the human body. Evil spirits can only enter the human body through persistent and wilful sinning, so to address all of this as if it were a piece of pure deliverance ministry can greatly increase ministry 'failure' rates as well as bringing the ministry into disrepute, and it does not honour our Lord. Suggesting that there may have been long periods of wilful sin in the life of the sufferer can easily lead either to hurtful rejection or sin–chasing on the part of the minister —both of which can do much harm.

However, some sickness is the result of demonic activity and should be treated as such. In such cases, the prime gift the minister needs to pray for is not the power to deliver but the grace to discern.

37. Is not everything in God's timing?

Out of a sense of pastoral care for those who have not been healed through our prayers, we sometimes fall back on the belief that 'It is all in God's timing!' It may be more truthful for us to tell the disappointed sufferer that we do not know why our prayers have not been answered; we cannot believe that God does not want to do it, so we guess (wrongly, of course) that because God is eternal, transcending time, he does not realise the urgency of the situation! And we know that a thousand years in his sight are like a day or a watch in the night (see Psalm 90:4), so we feel that all we can do is advise an unspecified time of waiting to see what will happen. In any case, the argument relieves the minister of any responsibility over the issue. However, we must keep our theology of healing as Christ–centred as we can, checking all the while with the words and works of Jesus before we philosophise about the nature of divine time.

The following passage is a clear indication of God's view of his timing when it applies to his healing work in the world.

> — and a man with a shrivelled hand was there. Looking for a reason to accuse Jesus, they asked him, "Is it lawful to heal on the Sabbath?"
>
> He said to them, "If any of you has a sheep and it falls into a pit on the Sabbath, will you not take hold of it and lift it out? How much more valuable is a man than a sheep! Therefore it is lawful to do good on the Sabbath." Then he said to the man, "Stretch out your hand." So he stretched it out and it was completely restored, just as sound as the other.
>
> *Matthew 12:10–13*

Some might have thought it prudent for Jesus to have asked the man with the withered hand to return the next day, so avoiding what was to be yet another confrontation between himself and the religious leaders of that time. But Jesus is demonstrating here that healing will not wait. His compassion will not allow any continuation of suffering. The sheep, in Jesus' example, cannot simply be left in the pit, for any reason. To imply that God does not care enough about our illnesses, and is prepared to let any amount of time pass by before he acts, does nothing but sow more doubt in the church. God's timing, quite simply, is *now*. 'Wait!' is not what Christ revealed. In healing the sick he always revealed the *'now!'* He did not teach us that the 'Wait!' was on God's side. The only 'Wait!' was self–imposed, applying to those people who did not come to Christ for healing. In the New Testament, in the matter of healing, if there is a 'Wait!', it is on the human side. Our attitude today should be that we must militantly pray, and receive all that Jesus has done. This may mean spiritual warfare and prevailing prayer until we receive. Anyone who believes that God sometimes may say 'Wait to be healed!' to them will have difficulty in being able to prevail in spiritual warfare and prayer. The idea creates doubt, and saps spiritual energy, reducing the supplicant's expectancy for healing, and it promotes passiveness and even more failure in ministry. Expectancy concerning Jesus Christ's willingness to heal is fundamental to prevailing, even if it does take a season to receive.

38. Is healing a special gifting?

Yes and no. Healing is a special gifting in that it flows continuously and wonderfully out of the merciful heart of God, and 'no' in the sense that no one individual can heal the sick without being in tune with the Holy Spirit and with the will of God to heal. The actual power is God's. Certain people may have other personality gifting which propels them to the centre of the stage of Christian life, but the actual kingdom healing power comes from God and him alone.

Every Christian can be used to heal the sick, as long as they are walking in the anointing to do so which has been given to the whole church. The anointing is on all of us —it is the walking into it and in it that is often missing.

Many believe that only some of us have gifts of healing to give to others because 1 Corinthians 12 appears to imply this, in contrast to the view expressed here that anyone in the church can bring sick and injured people into healing. There is a third dimension missing in this argument. Firstly, there are different gifts flowing through different people, but we need to recognize that many do not have the ability to see healing happen. This is because they have not, as yet, been taught how to do so. Any Christian, properly equipped, can see great increases in his or her effectiveness in any of the gifts listed by Paul. Healing is never a question of having some sort of holy talent; it is always a question of being able to raise the supplicant's expectant faith and to bring them into God's presence. This can be taught.

In Peter's address to the house of Cornelius we find six principles to adhere to in such an anointed walking.

> You know the message God sent to the people of Israel, telling the good news of peace through Jesus Christ, who is Lord of all. You know what has happened throughout Judea, beginning in Galilee after the baptism that John preached —how God anointed Jesus of Nazareth with the Holy Spirit and power, and how he went around doing good and healing all who were under the power of the devil, because God was with him.
>
> *Acts 10:36–38*

The six principles involved in living in kingdom healing anointing drawn from the above description of Jesus are:

1. '...How God anointed Jesus of Nazareth with the Holy Spirit and power.' It is of importance that we should continually be asking that we be filled with the Holy Spirit, as he is our Guide and pointer to Jesus.
2. '...And how he went around.' We may understand from this statement that Jesus did not merely sit and wait, praying for people and expecting all those who wanted him to find their own way to his side. We must expect to have to be 'out there' with the sick and the injured, taking risks with our faith, and giving all the credit and praise to God.
3. 'Doing good.' It is generally understood that this expression refers to the compassion of Jesus for the sick.

> A man with leprosy came to him and begged him on his knees, "If you are willing, you can make me clean."
>
> Filled with compassion, Jesus reached out his hand and touched the man. "I am willing," he said. "Be clean!"
>
> *Mark 1:40–41*

It is this compassion for those who suffer that is a major factor in seeing healing take place.

4. '...And healing all.' To consistently see healing and miracles taking place it is vital to believe that it is God's will to see everyone restored. This belief can be likened to our pushing a lightning conductor up into the sky, while any form of doubt is a pressure to pull it down again. Where the net result is positive, at least as large as a mustard seed, then we are able to receive, and help others to receive, kingdom healing.

5. '...Who were under the power of the devil.' For further reading, see No. 36 *Is it always the devil who wants us to be ill?*

6. '...Because God was with him.' Jesus taught that he and the Father are one. Jesus made it clear that he would indwell believers, and that the kingdom of God is within them. The power that raised Jesus from the dead is at work in Christians. We are a temple of the Holy Spirit. So no individual Christian can say that they do not have access to the power and authority to heal.

All six of these components should be in place and working together —not merely any one of them, according to the latest spiritual fashion trends. To walk effectively in the anointing to heal, not only should all six features be present in our ministry, we should be seeking to grow each one through our own Christian discipleship and openness to the Holy Spirit.

39. What about Paul's thorn in the flesh?

Of all the misgivings people articulate about God's willingness to heal the sick, Paul's thorn in the flesh is most often quoted. Despite Paul's praying three times, God told Paul that his grace was sufficient. It is thought that he would not heal him of some worrying complaint.

> To keep me from becoming conceited because of these surpassingly great revelations, there was given me a thorn in my flesh, a messenger of Satan, to torment me. Three times I pleaded with the Lord to take it away from me. But he said to me, "My grace is sufficient for you, for my power is made perfect in weakness." Therefore I will boast all the more gladly about my weaknesses, so that Christ's power may rest on me.
>
> *2 Corinthians 12:7–9*

But does this passage really provide evidence that God is sometimes reluctant to heal? There are several points to consider. Firstly, where one piece of Scripture seems to contradict all the rest it is always better to question our own understanding of it. Both the Old and the New Testament portray God as the healer of all our diseases, not the force instigating them, nor the force prolonging them. Secondly, the thorn is described as a messenger of Satan, sent to keep him from becoming conceited because of some surpassingly great revelations. The expression 'of Satan' only tells us that the messenger had an evil streak in their make–up. It would only be God who would wish to see Paul remaining in humility, and God is never the instigator of sickness. It is therefore extremely unlikely that the thorn was any sort of illness or deformity, as these things do not come from God. Thirdly, the thorn is described as a messenger; and this is a term used for a person, not a disease. Its purpose was to stop Paul from being big–headed, and sickness does not do that —whereas people might. Fourthly, Paul was a fine student and teacher of the Law. He knew his Hebraic history and all its writings.

> For you have heard of my previous way of life in Judaism, how intensely I persecuted the church of God and tried to destroy it. I was advancing in Judaism beyond many Jews of my own age and was extremely zealous for the traditions of my fathers.
>
> *Galatians 1:13–14*

Throughout the Old Testament we find references to thorns in the flesh that would have been well known to Paul. One early example is,

> "But if you do not drive out the inhabitants of the land, those you allow to remain will become barbs in your eyes and thorns in your sides. They will give you trouble in the land where you will live."
>
> *Numbers 33:55*

If it were an actual thorn, then Paul would not have had to resort to prayer to remove it. Clearly, thorns in the flesh are people who manipulate, control and otherwise plague our lives. Under such circumstances, would not the grace of God indeed be a strength, and sufficient for any of us?

There is yet another stream of thinking from those more minded towards spiritual warfare. The Greek word used here for messenger is 'angelos', a term used in the New Testament to signify a personal being, not an illness. Following the shipwrecks, beatings and imprisonments, it would not have surprised Paul that an angel of Satan had indeed been sent to plague him and attempted to block his activities.

This thorn is not a sickness but some unpleasant character or other, spiritual or human.

40. What about the kingdom being 'now, but not yet'?

The question of the kingdom being 'now but not yet' —here but not yet in its fullness—springs from a theological viewpoint held for many hundreds of years, namely that whilst the kingdom of God that was taught and displayed by Jesus is in a sense present here now, it has somehow not yet entirely come. An alternative view is that it did indeed come in fullness with Jesus, but has somehow dwindled away since his Ascension. Despite the power injected into the church at Pentecost, the ability either of God, or of modern–day Christian disciples, to perform miracles through his grace, has somehow degenerated to very little. Everything, we read in Scripture, has been placed under the feet of Jesus and yet we do not (as yet) see everything behaving as if it were so. It concludes that, one way or the other, this is because the kingdom is only partially here. Whilst we can accept that Father does want us well, we think of the second coming of Christ as the time and place at which the will of God will be visibly, completely fulfilled. This is the time when all will be healed. We will have to wait until then for full healing in body, mind and spirit. This view, which is sometimes advanced to account for the lack of healing in the church today, when put another way, entails the idea that God does not want to heal some of us. As some certainly do receive healing, then the idea of a 'weak' version of the finished kingdom presupposes that God is arbitrarily deciding on healing some and not others because his kingdom is somehow not powerful enough to heal everybody yet. A less objectionable explanation is that some are still not receiving because theological ideas like this are openly taught and promoted. Such ideas only serve to create doubt, and doubt is a potent barrier to receiving healing. If our expectancy is an important factor in healing, as Jesus' teaching and practice indicates, the last thing we need is doubt. Such ideas as 'now, but not yet...' lead us to think that healing might well not happen after prayer, and so our expectancy of God is reduced.

This theology of 'now, but not yet...' needs to be viewed from a very different angle. The question to hand should really be this: is the 'not yet' part because God is not giving us the kingdom completely, or is it simply because we are no longer equipped to understand and deal with things in the way Jesus would have done? Could it be that we do not see everything under Jesus' feet, not because, in a sense, that full authority has yet to be manifested, but rather because we have not yet learned to place everything there? What shall we do with such a verse as, "Do not be afraid, little flock, for your Father has been pleased to give you the kingdom" (Luke 12:32)?

God is completely reliable in all his promises, and is not giving the kingdom to us partially. Let us hold on to the undeniable fact that Jesus demonstrated, during his earthly ministry, that the expression of the kingdom on earth at that time was more than adequate to deal with every kind of illness and pain in everyone who came to him. The disciples who were sent out by Jesus, the apostles, and the other leaders in the early church, also seemed to be able to demonstrate this. The insinuation that, in this present day and age, the kingdom is somehow less here today than it was in Jesus' day is unbiblical and theologically problematic.

But, then, what has changed? —because something certainly seems to have done. We do not often see healing and miracles on the New Testament scale. We need to see that the problem is not on God's side of the kingdom but on the human side. On God's part, the work of the cross is complete. The kingdom is now present —and not in some sort of lesser and weaker way than it was in Jesus's time on earth. He was simply better at expressing God's kingdom than we seem to be. In fact, he was perfect at doing it! The first disciples may not have got it right every time, but the number of their 'failures' pales into insignificance, compared with the level of ministry failure apparent today. Today, those of us who are receiving and ministering healing in the kingdom have minds that are full of problems about both areas. We hear things that hinder our trust in Jesus and create doubt. This theology of the presence of a partial kingdom has deeply influenced our beliefs and ministry practices, and has therefore affected our experience. Jesus never taught this doctrine, it is of man's devising. 'Not yet' is not what Jesus revealed. He always revealed the 'now' in the doing of healing miracles. We should learn again from Jesus how to express the kingdom in the same way that he taught his first disciples to do, so that the sick around us will be healed.

41. Does God raise the dead?

There have been a few recorded cases of resurrection to life in recent years, but these are rare. Some are fully documented and vindicated by the medical profession. There are also a number of anecdotal stories around the church and, adding these all together, we can only give glory to God for his wonders. However, any suggestion that Jesus should or could raise every dead person whose relatives come to him and ask is clearly erroneous. If we keep our perspective Christ–centred, we will not find any evidence that might lead us to this conclusion. We know that Jesus repeatedly healed all the sick in the multitudes who came to listen to him and to be healed of their diseases, but there is nothing at all in Scripture on which to base the idea that Christ responded to every request for a resurrection. We do not even know if anyone asked him; no such requests are recorded. We can only consider the three resurrections Jesus carried out: the raising from death of Lazarus; the widow of Nain's son; and the synagogue official's daughter. There may have been many other such situations brought to Jesus' attention, yet only three stories are given. Does this demonstrate favouritism on God's part? Is his grace a random affair? Neither of these arguments hold water, as God shows no more love for one bereaved family than for another —all his love and attention is focused on each of us. There are other things to be discovered here. The raising of Lazarus demonstrates that Jesus is himself everlasting life, and that he was sent by the Father. (See John 11:41–42). The widow of Nain's son was raised as a demonstration of the power of God's compassion; and the story of the synagogue official's daughter shows us much about the necessity to create and preserve a faith environment, as far as possible unhindered by doubt, for a miracle to take place. (See Luke 8:50–51).

None of these three resurrection incidents in the Gospels records any direct requests from grieving relatives. Again, the somewhat thin evidence we might see in the disciples' request to Peter to 'Come at once!' in response to Tabitha's death, is not sufficient to enable us to determine anything definitive on this point.

> In Joppa there was a disciple named Tabitha (which, when translated, is Dorcas), who was always doing good and helping the poor. About that time she became sick and died, and her body was washed and placed in an upstairs room. Lydda was near Joppa; so when the

> disciples heard that Peter was in Lydda, they sent two men to him and urged him, "Please come at once!"
>
> Peter went with them, and when he arrived he was taken upstairs to the room. All the widows stood around him, crying and showing him the robes and other clothing that Dorcas had made while she was still with them. Peter sent them all out of the room; then he got down on his knees and prayed.
>
> Turning toward the dead woman, he said, "Tabitha, get up." She opened her eyes, and seeing Peter she sat up.
>
> *Acts 9:36–40*

We should note that the initial request was not specifically for a miracle of resurrection but simply for Peter's attendance at the grieving household. We might wish to make an assumption about what the disciples had in mind by such a request, but we cannot be certain. In today's ministry, it may be that the best advice is to avoid attempting such a miracle unless the immediate family have specifically requested it, and only then within a faith environment and where prayers may be said in faith by all concerned.

Part Five

Pastoral and Practical

42. What if my church is not yet ready for a healing ministry?

This question is often asked in relation to a congregation that knows little or nothing, or does not wish to know, about the Christian healing ministry. It is also used to explain away any personal experiences of unanswered prayer which may have left behind feelings of disappointment or rejection that cannot be admitted to in the face of God, who is good. It may also be an expression of doubt on the part of the church leadership.

Some believe that the power of the kingdom, as demonstrated by Jesus, has somehow drained away. The power is simply not, we might be led to believe, here any more. The doctrine of the sinking kingdom is not, however, based in anything that can be found in Scripture. However, this misunderstanding is a belief, sometimes accompanied by a good deal of wishful thinking, that, if we can get filled enough with the Holy Spirit, all will come right for us again and we will be able to heal the sick. Some believe that, when we reach the point when God considers the church to be ready, we shall just be able then to get on and heal the sick without recourse to any strategy or experience. As with the apostles, only our presence will be necessary in a hospital or in a sick room, for we will be full of the Holy Spirit and self will have been utterly laid aside. Meanwhile, as some will have it, there is much more than healing for us to explore in the kingdom, so we need not concern ourselves with this small aspect of the gospel that much. Such arguments completely disregard both Pentecost and Jesus' commission given to the church in Matthew 10:7–8,

> As you go, preach this message: 'The kingdom of heaven is near.' Heal the sick, raise the dead, cleanse those who have leprosy, drive out demons. Freely you have received, freely give.

Jesus does not describe the kingdom as being weak and draining away but 'near'. It was most certainly near enough in his 'day' to enable all who asked him to receive healing. To see what the Holy Spirit wants the Christian church to understand by kingdom living, we need to look at the ministry of Jesus. Whatever else we might think it should be like today, if we cannot find it in Jesus' teaching and ministry, then it is a product of something not as Christ–centred as it might be. Here is a typical example of the nature of daily kingdom living:

> Great crowds came to him, bringing the lame, the blind, the crippled, the mute and many others, and laid them at his feet; and he healed them. The people were amazed when they saw the mute speaking, the crippled made well, the lame walking and the blind seeing. And they praised the God of Israel.
>
> *Matthew 15:30–31*

One of the hallmarks of our living in the kingdom of God is that needy people, the sick and injured, are brought into healing. The reason for this is a simple one—the atmosphere in the kingdom of God is of restoration. To put it another way, signs and wonders are the natural outcome of apostolic teaching. The gospel cannot be fully taught without them.

> I will not venture to speak of anything except what Christ has accomplished through me in leading the Gentiles to obey God by what I have said and done—by the power of signs and miracles, through the power of the Spirit. So from Jerusalem all the way around to Illyricum, I have fully proclaimed the gospel of Christ.
>
> *Romans 15:18–19*

God considered the time to be ready at Calvary, sending his Son to die, that power from heaven might be released into his people on earth. Pentecost, the point at which he sent his Spirit into the heart of the church, enabled the early Christians to have wonderfully productive healing ministries, to a level rarely seen today. It is not the kingdom that has weakened so drastically over the centuries, it is our trust in the King. We are not waiting for God—he is waiting for us.

For further reading see No. 40 *What about the kingdom being 'now, but not yet'?* And No. 38 *Is healing a special gifting?*

43. Could I get involved and minister healing to the sick?

> '...They will place their hands on sick people, and they will get well'
>
> *Mark 16:18b*

In this one simple, staggering, inspiring sentence, Jesus Christ tells the world something amazing about his disciples then and throughout the ages which were still to come. They could heal the sick! They did not have any particular medical ability of their own—the authority and the power came from God—but they took the initiative and saw results. "Lord," said the seventy-two, returning with joy from their teaching and healing mission, "even the demons submit to us in your name."

Doubters say that all those times have passed, but what happens if we do not want to doubt —if we want to follow Jesus in his ministry and help others, extending the kingdom of God and healing illness? What happens if we express a desire to heal the sick and to take joy in the results, as those early disciples did? Can we delight our heavenly Father and bring him pleasure by imitating his Son in healing the sick? Praying for people is one thing, but actually seeing them healed —that is quite another! Would it not be wonderful if it were true, that we could do such things today? Other than the re–building of the broken temple walls of body, mind and spirit, what else is there in this life to be so enthusiastic about —exciting enough to throw one's whole life into it? What lifts the soul into such passion to see the sufferer free? What is it that makes the heartbeat stumble a little with anticipation at the very thought of it? The answer to these questions lies waiting for us in the imagination of the soul. Such flurries of the heart, such love–passion to see his glory fall, these sensations occur as our own spirits leap towards our God, greater and more encompassing than the universe itself, and yet stooping to touch an individual soul with the healing tip of a finger. And touch us he surely does! When we consider God's mighty creation of the universe, of heaven and earth and the moon and the planets and stars he has placed above our heads, we have little option but to wonder at how precious to him we human beings must be, or how divine love has stooped to meet us. We can be assured that God is infinitely loving and caring toward each of us. His will for us is that we should be healed of all sickness and disease. He has made us only a little lower than the heavenly beings and crowned us with glory and honour. Compared with this generosity of God, what on this earth could mankind be, that the living God should make so much of us and pour out his love on us?

What can we know, then, of Jesus Christ, from our own experiences? We can know that he is alive, personal and real, and closer than we think. We may feel his presence. Many have felt his healing touch, and have seen the changes he has made in our lives, not just in lifting a mood or two, but in dissolving away confusion and doubt, melting our pride and persuading us to do the right thing —in other words, to be obedient. Most thrilling of all is the sight of him, or rather the strong and gentle effect of his power, as it brings his healing touch to huge numbers of people.

If we allow Jesus to reign in us, the Fatherhood of God is supreme, and we experience that as a living reality, not just a theological theory. We belong to him for we have become his children by adoption and grace, when we accepted Jesus as Saviour and Lord, turning to him in repentance, receiving him and accepting his sacrificial death on the cross as the price paid for our sins and our healing. Without him we would be absolutely powerless to do what we know we ought to do, to change our own character, habits or disposition, or to work with him to heal the sick. But he can change these things.

Aware of our own inadequacies, we learn of the power that

raised Jesus Christ from the dead that is now at work within us. We learn and experience his ability to change that which we are not able to change, providing of course that we are obedient to his leading.[1]

Could the reader get involved? Definitely! There will be much to learn and probably even more to unlearn. The road is sometimes rocky but it has the most wonderful views!

[1]Extract from *The Passion to Heal* by Mike Endicott

44. How should we prepare the congregation?

Our first step is to accept the church situation as it is at the moment, to look unblinkingly at the reality of it and, at the same time, to open our hands to accept willingly whatever our loving Father puts there.

Many express concern, if not frustration, because their leaders or other members of their congregation do not appear to desire a healing ministry. There is sometimes a note of embarrassment attached to this concern; a feeling of being let down, or worrying about what other members of the church may think if we broach the subject to them, corporately or even individually. Added to this, most flock leaders will also carry great fears of public failure and the consequent loss of trusting and obedient relationship between flock and shepherd.

There is a danger created by these concerns: that the would–be healing minister may become preoccupied with such issues, preventing them from fully appreciating their own relationship with, and knowledge of, God's kingdom and opening their hands to accept willingly however our loving Father leads.

If we find that we have no power to prevail over some

church situation, then we must leave it to God and allow our relationship with him to bloom. Should we even try to project onto leader or congregation our views and opinions about how a church ministry of healing might begin? Could this damage that relationship? What should we do if faced with the situation where the others seem uninterested in the ministry? Certainly we must leave it to God but, in doing so, we are doing more than we may think. By attending church, blossoming in our relationship with God, and not trying to persuade, manipulate or control anyone, but going simply and quietly about the business of encouraging the sick and injured to receive healing as we find them, we are then offering the strongest message of all —that of example. Example is not the main thing in influencing others—it is the only thing. If we try to influence one person by being a good example, we are usually influencing more than two. If we try to influence someone without being a good example, then we will not influence anyone. If we want our church leaders or congregation to see what Christ will do for them *en masse*, let them see what Christ has done for only one among them.

The healing ministry was not created by the church for something on which to ponder or to do in mission, but rather it is part of the taste of the outpouring of Christ into a rough and suffering world. It is not a ministry of the discussion forum but a ministry of ordinary, Christian rolled–up sleeves in the community. If we are to stand in the flow of healing mercy which is the selfless outpouring of Jesus, then we need to stand between him and the desperate who have, as yet, not found the river that flows from the high King of heaven.

We would best not discuss healing ministry at all, or struggle with opinions about how we might persuade the congregation towards our way of thinking, but to take such faith as we have in both hands, stand with the Word of God and the name of Jesus in our mouths, and simply *do* it.

Before we spend too much time, as leaders or healing

ministers, discussing how we might bend the opinions of our congregations to our own ways of thinking about healing, we might consider getting out into homes and hospitals and praying with the members who are sick there. In this way we face little or no argument and kingdom work is done in the meantime. In this fashion, and because we ourselves are members of our church, we bring a working ministry alive. It is always better to do it than to talk about it!

45. How do I teach healing effectively?

Boldness is the only way, and boldness is full of risk. Preaching the kingdom of God in relationship to his healing grace is necessarily difficult, as the New Testament does not give us precise enough definitions against which to teach the restorative nature of its atmosphere.

Therefore it would be better to teach about the King. Unless we teach of Jesus who gives healing to all who come, we will be teaching a different 'Jesus' than the one in the Gospels. Teaching about the One revealed in Scripture raises expectancy and builds the necessary faith environment, both around and within the preacher, for healing to happen.

It is also essential that we address the sort of everyday doubts that afflict the Christian mind, doubt being the force that is so obstructive of healing, as it reduces expectancy. One teaching pattern worth the examination would be that of Elijah on Mount Carmel. His first priority was to build an altar, and this can be done today by preaching Jesus as faithful and reliable Saviour, healer and Lord. There arises at this point another obvious requirement: the preacher, on his or her own part, has to believe it absolutely. In the taunting of the opposition and in the watering of his own sacrifice, Elijah deliberately set out to address the doubt of the unbelievers. The result was staggering. The people's doubt and unbelief was forcibly squashed by Elijah's down–to–earth comments, and the fire came from God. Elijah did not waste time with a long theological treatise, neither did he soften and fudge any part of the issue to make his message more palatable to those who might struggle with it. He spoke simply and precisely. In the same way, when we preach Jesus as the ultimately reliable healer, and talk in common sense ways to address people's doubts, we make it easier for them to receive healing.

To reflect on Elijah's marvellous example of expectancy in action is to learn something of how God wants his ministers to exercise faith in their proving demonstration of the kingdom. He did not climb Mount Carmel to pray for the people. He did not just offer to put king Ahab on his prayer list. He did not invite eight hundred and fifty false prophets to go up with him simply to preach to them. He took them to see the power of the living God.

46. Does this sort of healing last?

"Will the healing last? I will reserve judgement until I see how things are tomorrow!" Initial gains in physical and emotional healing may be lost at a later time. This is not the usual case, by any means, but it can happen within minutes (or perhaps a few days) after ministry.

Four broad types of reaction to the apparent loss of a divine gift of healing are common. Firstly, we may adopt the 'I told you so' approach, in which we vindicate negative thoughts that Christian healing might be mostly a question of wishful thinking. We wonder if we felt some improvement only because of some hype being experienced at a healing service, and maybe our apparent gain was simply the exercise of mind over matter. Either way, if the symptoms return, our scepticism is fortified. Secondly, we may begin to blame the speaker at the service or at the conference meeting at which we received some healing. Although he or she may never have claimed that anyone other than Jesus works miracles like these today, we dismiss them as 'charlatans'. What they were saying could not have been true after all. Thirdly, we may wonder if there might be something wrong with our faith, that has come into play after receiving a miracle blessing. Perhaps it was not as strong as we thought it was, or perhaps God discovered some underlying sin of which we were not aware, and so withdrew his blessing. Fourthly, most common, and most disastrous of all, is a sense of rejection by God. Any one of these four broad categories of thought pattern serves to reduce our expectancy of God and, in doing so, reduces our ability to receive any further.

So how can we seem to lose something that God has given? In Mark 4:4–8, Jesus gives a full explanation of these losses in the story of a farmer who went out to scatter seed.

> As he was scattering the seed, some fell along the path, and the birds came and ate it up. Some fell on rocky places, where it did not have much soil. It sprang up quickly, because the soil was shallow. But when the sun came up, the plants were scorched, and they withered because they had no root. Other seed fell among thorns, which grew up and choked the plants, so that they did not bear grain. Still other seed fell on good soil. It came up, grew and produced a crop, multiplying thirty, sixty, or even a hundred times.

Jesus then interprets the seed as being symbolic of the Word of God. We know that the Word made flesh is Christ himself, and that he is the perfect image of God, whose will is for all to receive healing. We can see by observing the whole earthly ministry of Jesus that the kingdom (the farm in the story) is a place of renewal, restoration, redemption and resurrection. We then notice here that, in the kingdom, it is God who sows the healing. Interestingly enough, it is in fact broadcast: scattered freely and openly and not put precisely in any chosen place as it would be with modern agricultural seed–drills. Healing is not a chosen and directed gift; it is a river of mercy that flows. Sometimes the seed falls on well–trodden and unyielding soil. The path is the way that so many of us go, believing that we know what there is to know and how we should rightly go about getting it. Our human knowledge, intellectual judgements, traditions, understandings and preferences make infertile ground. This leaves the seed exposed on the surface of our lives and the devil soon snatches it away, sometimes even before we can receive it. Other healing may fall on shallow soil, mixed with many stones, which themselves represent our doubts and cynical thoughts. Healing clings to our expectancy of God and doubts subtract from this fertility. Our healing springs up, but our expectancy and persistence in pursuing and keeping it are not strong enough to maintain the healing. Then there are the thorn bushes, other cares and influences of the world that throttle the mercy we have received. Doubting thoughts may crowd in from sceptical family and church alike. On the other hand we may become aware of the necessity for new lifestyle changes which we were not prepared for. There are many possible choking influences.

Gloriously, much seed falls on fertile ground where simple, child–like hearts have quietly taken hold of it. The good soil is our expectancy that God will do it for us, and there are few stones of doubt and scepticism to cause problems for the new plant. Such plants grow and flourish, and in turn may produce their own seed, which often goes on to bring about much healing in the lives of others.

Healing is always given, seed is always sown. The sower does not have to select the precise spot on the ground where each seed lands, nor does he remove some of the seed after the sowing. It is not the sower or the seed that we are to affect, it is simply the fertility of the ground that needs to benefit from our own attentions and efforts.

47. What about other forms of spiritual healing?

Sometimes the question is posed in this form: "Where I come from, people believe that the witch doctor can heal. When they have ailments, they go to see him and numbers of them get healed. How can this be?" Similar questions may be asked by those who have been involved with other forms of occult, psychical and spiritualist activity.

If the kingdom of God reacts in healing to those who respond to the good news of Jesus Christ, then how do people get healed in faiths where Jesus is not recognised as the Son of God, our Lord, Saviour and healer? This question could, guardedly in this context, be considered in the light of the fact that healing is a part of our salvation. Salvation is a generic term for a number of individual benefits at God's disposal —true peace and eternal life instead of punishment and eternal death; abundance instead of poverty; a share in Jesus' resurrection life; a new nature exchanged for the old one; and healing. All these things which were bound together on Calvary in the death of Jesus, by the grace of the Father, are included in the term 'salvation'. For deeper understanding of this, see No. 34 *Is healing in the atonement?*

Many of us are used to thinking of salvation only as being the resurrection, on the list above, but it is much more. However, each individual aspect, and in this case we are considering healing, can be best seen in the light of the promise of everlasting life, which flows from the atonement. We know that everlasting life in heaven is available to all by the grace of God, and we know that Jesus himself is the judge of all things, determining who shall or shall not enter. His judgement will grant that honour to anyone he chooses. For those who have accepted Jesus as Lord and Saviour, that entrance to heaven is guaranteed. Similarly, Jesus has long ago granted healing to anyone in need of it and it is not for us to make the decision for him about any individual case, or the method through which he works. Accepting Christ as healer does make receiving very much easier, just as accepting him as Lord and Saviour guarantees everlasting life with him. Anyone may come to Jesus and expect to receive healing. When the multitudes came to Jesus for healing, he is certainly not depicted as checking out their orthodoxy before healing them!

There is great danger, on the other hand, in approaching other supernatural forces and, very often, a big price to pay. A large warning must be posted here. There are many forces abroad in the world which are opposed to Jesus Christ. For this reason, the God of Abraham, Isaac and Jacob is a jealous God, and abhors our approaching the spirits of dead people, our ancestors, or any spirit (claiming to have been medically trained during earthly existence or otherwise), that we might be tempted to believe may be kindly disposed towards us. The range of deceptions on offer is vast. God has been quite clear in his instructions about this.

> When you enter the land the LORD your God is giving you, do not learn to imitate the detestable ways of the nations there. Let no one be found among you who sacrifices his son or daughter in the fire, who practices divination or sorcery, interprets omens, engages in witchcraft, or casts spells, or who is a medium or

> spiritist or who consults the dead. Anyone who does these things is detestable to the LORD, and because of these detestable practices the LORD your God will drive out those nations before you. You must be blameless before the LORD your God.
>
> *Deuteronomy 18:9–13*

Again, Pharaoh's magicians were found to be quite capable of throwing down their own sticks and making snakes of them, just as Moses had done shortly before, in the course of his attempts to free the children of Israel. The symbolism of the result should not escape us: Moses' snake gobbled up those of the magicians. Medical science can only be seen as a gift to us from God, but any supernatural healing coming from anyone or any organisation which does not acknowledge Jesus Christ as the only Lord, Saviour and healer does not come from him. Any other world religion, the occult and any of the wide variety of new age sources would all fit into this classification. The deceiving power behind these faiths and 'spiritual' activities is the 'god of this world', and the devil will do works through his erring servants which give the appearance of being 'good'.

Logic dictates that, as the cause of some sickness is demonic activity, the enemy can temporarily remove the symptoms to fool the unwary. His motive for doing things like this is to keep us tied into false belief systems which will not eternally save us. He counterfeits many things, healing among them.

Jesus came to save the whole world, not just good church people. Healing is part of that salvation. Unlikely people will be saved and likely people may not be. We are not to be the judges in individual cases. God's plan is the salvation of the whole world through Jesus and, therefore, receiving and abiding in Jesus, as Lord, Saviour and healer guarantees salvation, both in this world and the next.

48. Can I not just pray at a distance?

It would be much easier to sit quietly somewhere and pray for the sick. Alone in prayer we do not have to face any unbeliefs and misunderstandings. In the kingdom of God there is an atmosphere entirely made up of love so pure that it is beyond our imagining. That love is so vibrant and passionate that, sharper than any double–edged sword, it longs to penetrate deep into our souls and spirits, joints and marrow, measuring the thoughts and attitudes of our hearts. The power of it is so intense that it heals the sick. This energetic atmosphere of power love passes into the world through the hands and lives of Christians —those who both live in the kingdom and have expectant faith in Jesus; and healing and wholeness are brought into people's lives as part of their salvation while they still live and suffer in the world. At the end of life, kingdom living guarantees passage into everlasting bliss with the God who reigns in heaven.

Living the kingdom life on earth is not a soft option to choose. It is not a soothing retreat from the difficulties of everyday life, more like an invitation to three things. First, we are being asked to enter fully into this problematic life, to apply there the grace and the mercies of the King himself, and bear the cost of doing so. When Jesus taught us to pray, he encouraged us to look away from the everyday world in which we are distracted by what we see and feel, instead opening our hearts and spirits to God. Even so, he always demonstrated that our faith must be related to life 'in the raw'. It is only through our constant prayer contact with the King that a better quality of kingdom living can be achieved. Jesus himself spent many hours in communion with the Father, and then showed us that this new quality of life has to be both tested and demonstrated in the ordinary rough–and–tumble of plain living. Our model must be Jesus, the healing King of the disciple's life in the workplace, on the roads, in the crowded shopping mall, facing vociferous demands and quarrelsome opposition, amid the lack of much private life and amongst all the untimely interruptions to our well–planned and orderly lives; he is to be Lord of all these areas, as well as our crucified Saviour who died for us that we might have life. All this is not merely like, but is in reality, the divine life operating under human conditions, and it underlines the true validity and necessity of our communion with God even in our ordinary and everyday human relationships. Without this—the very real and practical operation of love—theological exactitude is not worth much at all. Set against this picture of the kingdom, distractions like church power politics look as childish as they really are. In comparison to true kingdom living, such so–called 'ministries' as the politically correct posturing of the Righteously Indignant, and those in need of having their egos massaged, do not look at all like the ministry of Jesus.

In the light of the true magnificence of the kingdom and all its works, our own sinfulness, while it cannot be ignored, pales into relative insignificance while the mystery of God is all around us, and our souls bloom in all their fullest colour. In the context of this kingdom of God there is little point in talking about love unless we are prepared to 'do' it. We cannot simply assume that people know that God loves them, or that we are concerned about them, or that we want to help by ministering to them the signs and the wonders of the kingdom. If we merely stay sitting in our pews, whispering prayers for them but never making a move in their direction they may never know what God's healing love really is.

We need the holy courage to approach those in trouble and say, 'What can I do to help?' Many of us have had the uncomfortable experience of being drawn this way into other people's bottomless pits, but when fear of saying the wrong thing or risking another bottomless pit stands in the way of our ministering to others, then we have lost sight of God's purpose. We are not being, for others, a sign of Christ. Such fears are enemies of the kingdom, yet the kingdom is supposed to be in the middle of our enemies. Those of us who take the conscious decision not to suffer in this way do not fully want to be of the kingdom of Jesus; we may rather be among friends, sitting in the sunshine of the social life among roses and soft furnishings, not with uncomfortable sickness but in spiritual huddles with our other devout friends. This is a betrayal of the lifestyle of Christ.

49. What about the laying on of hands?

The laying on of hands and the anointing with oil are often seen as being sacramental acts, that is to say, the outward and visible signs of inward and invisible graces. We may add to those two things the use of prayer cloths, the lying under Peter's shadow (both biblical acts), the later use of touching with reliquaries and even our attendance at such places as Lourdes today. Acts of Jesus himself might add to this list the pushing of fingers into the ears of the hard of hearing, the spitting in the face of the visually impaired, the application of a mixture of spittle and clay and touching the tongues of those with speech impediments. The example of Elisha might even demand the dipping of leprous skin in the river Jordan. Some of these are familiar accounts of outward signs of pending inward grace. The real question is, do these things work, or are they merely meaningless ritual?

A single common denominator underlies 'sacramental acts' —they lift the supplicant's expectancy that God will act. It may be that, with the passage of the centuries of church life, some may be guilty of reaching a place where the outward sacramental act is relied upon to do the work, rather than real expectancy of God to open us to his wonders. This is the point at which an act becomes mere ritual. To see the sick consistently being healed, we need to set up two things: we need to see them surrounded in a faith environment, and we need to pray in faith ourselves. Biblically warranted sacramental acts, like the laying–on–of–hands, if used in support of the faith environment, can provide great encouragement. It is generally considered that such acts, of themselves, do not carry any intrinsic power from God, but, when used to lift expectancy in the supplicant, they can be a powerful tool in the kingdom.

50. What are partial healings and why do they happen?

A partial healing occurs when healing has been received but not to the level and depth that is wished for, either by the minister or by the supplicant. The normal reaction may be disappointment, but that would be very wrong; disappointment tends to breed doubt; and then, too often and quite wrongly, God is supposed either to be incapable of doing the healing or only willing to do half the job. This cannot be a true picture of the heart of God to heal, as Jesus himself, on one occasion only, first carried out a partial healing but then went on to completion.

> They came to Bethsaida, and some people brought a blind man and begged Jesus to touch him. He took the blind man by the hand and led him outside the village. When he had spit on the man's eyes and put his hands on him, Jesus asked, "Do you see anything?"
>
> He looked up and said, "I see people; they look like trees walking around." Once more Jesus put his hands

on the man's eyes. Then his eyes were opened, his sight was restored, and he saw everything clearly.

Mark 8:22–25

The eventual ending of this story shows us that God's heart is to see full restoration. So why do partial healings happen? Three keys are necessary to release healing in the supplicant, keys which involve the minister, the supplicant and the surrounding body of Christ at prayer. They are expectancy, persistence and humility. Often the major difficulty is lack of persistence; that is, at least, the best place to start looking. In the passage quoted above, Jesus demonstrates that full healing often comes through persistent ministry. Had he given thanks for the condition of seeing men that look like trees, and then sent the man home with some encouragement to be thankful for small mercies, then his sight might never have been fully restored. Lack of persistence is a major cause of half–success. Even when the supplicant has sky–high expectancy, and is prepared to be persistent, full healing may not be received. In these cases it is always worth continuing another day, as something indefinable often changes within the supplicant, or within the minister, that makes all the difference. This time of tension often releases deep doubts that need to be dealt with.

As ministers we must be careful not to pre–judge the supplicant's needs. Sometimes they may only want, for example, sufficient strength to continue life as it is. Sometimes they are too frightened of the social, economic or stress changes that could occur if full healing were to be received. In other words, full healing is often, and somewhat mistakenly, a measure made by the minister and not by the supplicant. God's grace is to will healing for the supplicant to the level of their expectancy, or, put another way, God does not force healing on anyone, even if the minister would like to see it.

When he had gone indoors, the blind men came to him, and he asked them, "Do you believe that I am able to do this?"

"Yes, Lord," they replied.

Then he touched their eyes and said, "According to your faith will it be done to you."

Matthew 9:28–29

Our level of expectancy should be raised by a partial healing, not diminished by it. Seeing it, we should rejoice that it is a demonstration that the kingdom is near and that God is showing his willingness to heal. It should be an encouragement to us to go on persistently, to the level of the supplicant's wishes. The blessings of partial healing are not occasions for despair but are signs pointing forward in hope.

51. Should I stop taking the medicine?

Understanding that, in Jesus's teaching, faith plays a major part in the healing process, many people question whether continuing with a prescribed course of medicine after prayer will display a lack of faith in the heavenly realms, and whether, therefore, God might reduce, or not bring to completion, their healing. It is as though to continue taking medical treatment displays doubt, the opposite of trust in the King.

This is not a biblical principle. In the time of Jesus' ministry on earth, it was the priesthood, operating under the law of Moses, who had authority to adjudicate as to whether or not anyone was now well, following a period of serious illness. The decision was theirs, not that of the supplicant. So Jesus encourages healed people to re–visit the medical authority, in those days the priest, to have the healing properly authenticated. (See Luke 5:12–14). The leper making the sacrifice for cleansing would demonstrate to the priest the supplicant's total belief in his healing, thus keeping his expectancy alive until the healing was fulfilled.

Many healings take place over time. Much medical treatment is designed to support us while healing (natural or divine, if we wish to distinguish between them) carries on to completion. It would be foolish to take away that support which may be needed in the healing process.

In our bodies we have many mechanisms for natural healing, and that is how God intended it to be. The created order is his creation, though marred by man's disobedience and 'enemy activity'. So, when we read in the Gospels of those many miracles Jesus worked, we see divine power at work. What we might categorise as 'natural' or 'supernatural', in God's economy are not as distinct as we might think, for he is Lord over all —the 'natural' world and those special events that we call miracles.

Professional opinion authenticating a healing can be beneficial for the supplicant, and releases more praise, through him or her, to the glory of God.

52. Should we seek to heal all the sick we become aware of: the complete stranger limping down the street, for example, or everyone in the local hospital?

Firstly, the results would probably be very disappointing. Secondly, we must follow the example of Jesus in order to keep our ministry Christ–centred. If the giving of gifts of healing were entirely under the control of the person who has the gift, then it would be possible to heal everyone we want to. However, the New Testament makes it clear that healing nearly always involves either expectancy in the person being prayed for, or expectancy, persistence and humility in a relative, friend or someone else. The proactive healing approach may well not work because there might not be a faith environment around the sick person. Without such an environment we cannot expect even a mustard seed of expectancy to be raised, and kingdom healing is a response to the healing King. In the majority of the recorded miracles in the Gospels, the supplicant, or his friends and relatives, are responding in some simple and child–like way to either the words or the works of Jesus and, in doing so, they are stepping into this faith environment. Those who did not respond did not receive healing. (See Matthew 18:3 and 19:14.)

The passage in John's Gospel that describes the actions of Jesus at the pool of Bethesda (5:6–8) is sometimes quoted as a justification for proactive, rather than reactive, healing ministry to the sick and injured. However, two things are apparent in this passage. Firstly, Jesus is engaging the would–be supplicant in conversation about his difficulties. The sick man does not waste time describing at length his condition and its disadvantages, but expresses only a desperation to find some way of being released from his situation. The very fact that a teacher of the Law would be this interested at such a private level would have raised the man's interest. Recognised ministers of the church today may sometimes find that their 'rank' alone will carry sufficient authority to raise hopes. Secondly, Jesus uses a military command to address him: 'Get up!' Such a command, delivered with his firm authority, would have been enough to create around him a faith environment as big (or as small) as a mustard seed —sufficient to see the kingdom working. So what about the others? What about the rest of the disabled people scattered around the pool and waiting for their cure? Did Jesus simply turn his back on them? Did he pick out of the crowd the one that was going to be easy? This cannot be the case, as we know that God is not in any way selective about how he distributes his love among his children. We know also that Jesus is the only perfect revelation of our Father in heaven, and that his obedience to the Father's will was total. We do know, however, that lack of expectancy, described biblically as doubt and unbelief, keeps healing away. The only people in the New Testament who were not healed of their sicknesses were those who either stayed away from Jesus or did not believe in him, even to mustard seed proportions. There is also an underlying sense, in the various forms of the Great Commission, that healing itself is not the end product, but a sign pointing to Jesus and the wonder of the King working in the kingdom. So our duty as Christians is to spread the good news of the kingdom as our first outreach priority, and to do that in such a way that those hearing us find the healing power therein. It would be better that we share our faith with others as, if what comes out of us is apostolic teaching, then miracles of power will naturally follow on in proof of what we are saying.

53. What about internet and email prayer chains?

These are modern and popular technological methods used to involve as many as possible in praying for those who are sick or troubled within the community. One message about a sick person can easily and efficiently involve huge numbers of people in praying. One prayer request could be in a thousand different homes in seconds. When a loved one is suffering, it is hard to avoid the temptation of believing that numbers are important. It seems that the bigger the prayer chain the better. The more who know of the problem, the more clamour there will be in heaven. The reverse thought can be present as well: if we do not have access to a prayer chain we may feel somehow hopeless and disempowered. Because Jesus and Peter dismissed doubters from their presence (when dealing with the raising of the dead) it is sometimes believed that the general emailing of prayer requests might actually bring doubters into the prayer group, and therefore reduce the chances of a healing taking place. This latter argument cannot be valid, as prayer chains and email lists of intercessors are, by their very nature, disembodied organisations: if they are a community, that would be in a very attenuated sense —they can only be a community of individuals. Actually, the numbers involved in healing prayer make no difference at all. Levels of expectancy and persistence make all the difference in the world. We might have a thousand on our mailing list but it is only the faith of the expectant one that will prevail. Elijah, after all, was only a man just like us. He was only one person but his prayer was mighty and effective. (See James 5:17–18.) The overall view expressed in the Bible is that as many as possible should be gathered together for the purposes of worship, but this emphasis is not present in connection with the subject of intercession. It could be said that there were occasions in the Gospels where 'four', or 'they', or 'some people' brought a sick person to Jesus, but the biblical emphasis in these passages lies on the acts of healing and perhaps on the role of faith in the process, but not on the numbers who brought the supplicant.

In James 5:14, we read that if any one of us should fall ill we should inform the elders of the church and ask them to pray over us and anoint us with oil in the name of the Lord. There is a real sense here that being together with the elders as they pray is a vital part of the ministry, rather than distance praying. We are not being asked to inform them so that they may pray for us *in absentia*. It is the prayer offered in expectancy which will make the sick person well, rather than the number of elders present.

•

For further reading see No. 48 *Can I not just pray at a distance?*

54. When we finish our ministry to an individual, what should we then do about them?

The temptation will be to let go of them. We may justify this course of action by telling ourselves that we have done everything we can, that it is all in God's hands now, but we should be most careful that we are not exhibiting our own lack of trust. After all, to go back again to the person and ask them how they are is really putting one's faith on the line. They may not have been able to receive any healing at all, and we fear being left with egg on our faces and without the wisdom to take the next step. After we have ministered to the supplicant, one of three things will have happened: full or partial healing, or no apparent healing at all. Can we help any further? We need to remember the need for persistence in ministry balanced against the perceived threat of disappointment and our own pastoral concerns for the supplicant's faith.

The ministry of healing has been given to us to discharge —things are not all in God's hands now, they are still in ours. The greatest blockage to our receiving healing (and the only one in the New Testament) is our doubts. Good pastoral care would surely not be to let go but to see if there is a way to helping the supplicant realise, and then overcome, their doubts. The more we overcome these doubts the more we open ourselves to receiving healing. Anyone properly prepared in the healing ministry to the sick and injured ought to be able to fulfil this role to a great extent. We can at least offer 'counselling' where we may gently prise open the supplicant's doubts, but we had better be sure of the biblical answers and our concrete theology of healing before we do, otherwise they will not be helped. We have to ensure, as far as we may, that their expectancy minus their doubts still leaves them with a mustard seed of trust in Jesus as healer.

Jesus is our perfect example in ministry. He healed a man born blind on the Sabbath, and after much enquiry and argument the authorities threw him (the healed man) out of the Temple.

> To this they replied, "You were steeped in sin at birth; how dare you lecture us!" And they threw him out.
>
> Jesus heard that they had thrown him out, and when he found him, he said, "Do you believe in the Son of Man?"
>
> *John 9:34–35*

Jesus heard what was going on and went looking for him. Again, in the story of the Good Samaritan Jesus underlines our need to see the job to completion. In swallowing all our pride and going back to seek out the supplicant we display into the heavens humility, persistence and expectancy of God, the three major ingredients for receiving healing. Where numbers or geography make such searching out impracticable, public notice of our availability for further prayer and discussion must be made. Our underlying ministry tone must never be 'hit and run', but 'how can we serve you more?'